SOS: TMJ RESCUE
Don't Be Deceived...Your Symptoms are REAL!

Foreword: Noah S. Siegel, MD
Introduction: Jamison R. Spencer, DMD, MS

By Dr. Hitesh Patel

Dedication

To Beena, Rishi, Bindi, Ameet, Ryaan, and Neil who have inspired me with the true meaning and purpose of life, love, and understanding. They have given me life's greatest blessing and have helped me make a positive difference in people's lives.

Acknowledgments

The book would not have been possible without the support and encouragement of my mentors and colleagues. There are many people who have helped me with this book.

A profound thank you to Dr. Jamison Spencer for his generous mentorship and sharing of knowledge and expertise. Thank you to Dr. Michael Goldberg for his hours of help with editing and assistance in conveying my thoughts into words.

I am honored Dr. Noah Siegel penned the forward to this book. Dr. Seigel is a respected physician in Boston who is Boarded in Otolaryngology and Sleep Medicine.

Many of my esteemed colleagues, part of an amazing Elite Mastermind in the Spencer Study Club, were essential in their input in the various chapters of the book, thank you to all of you:

Dr. Amy Thompson, Dr. Ashley Smitherman,
Dr. Carmine Morreale, Dr. Chiarina Iregui, Dr. Chuck Jelinek,
Dr. Claire-Marie Bender, Dr. Elizabeth Duling, Dr. Erica Johannes
Dr. Frank Henrich, Dr. Gemma Kwolek,
Dr. Jessica Sabo, Dr. Joan Werleman, Dr. John Kim,
Dr. Kathi Wilson, Dr. Keith Valachi, Dr. Kevin Postol,
Dr. Kip Covington, Dr. Sharnell Muir, and Dr. Tanya Kushner

And last but not least, thank you to Jenni Spencer and the entire Spencer team who, alongside their renowned "Commander in Sleep" Dr. Jamison Spencer, work tirelessly towards educating both health professionals and the public on the importance of a healthy night's sleep.

Editor in Chief—Jennifer Spencer
Assistant Editor—Dr. Michael Goldberg

Table of Contents

Table of Contents 4

Foreword 7

Introduction 9

1
TMJ, The Great Imposter 13

2
It's Not All in Your Head 22

*Even Though It's Not All in Your Head,
What IS in Your Head
Can Make a Huge Difference!* 22

3
"I've Got TMJ!" 26

The Most Amazing Joint in the Body! 26

4
**Chewing is Awesome!
(When It Doesn't Hurt)** 32

*The Muscles of Mastication
& How We Chew* 32

5
Lips Together, Teeth Apart 43

*The Best Way to Avoid & Treat
Many TMJ Problems
(Easier Said Than Done)* 43

6
Yes, Stress Can Cause Clenching & Grinding, But So Can… 48

*Medications and Other Things that
Contribute to Clenching & Grinding* 48

7
**Clenching & Grinding Your Teeth
Might Cause…** 56

8
But Wait There's More! 60

Other Things Clenching & Grinding Might Cause 62

9
What's That Popping & Clicking? 66

A Guide to the Common Noises in the Jaw Joint 66

10
When the Clicking STOPS… That's Probably Bad 73

Do You Have a Closed Lock? 73

11
TMJ X-Rays & Imaging 76

What to Expect from a Patient's Perspective 76

12
Who Needs to Be Treated? 80

The PDQ Method 80

13
Treating Muscle Pain & Headaches 87

The Most Common "TMJ Problem" 87

14
You Probably Don't Have a Botox Deficiency 92

15
Sprains Aren't Just for Ankles 98

Ligament & Tendon Issues 98

16
Treating Popping & Clicking 105

Why a Dental Term Called "Centric Relation" is Important to you 105

17
Your Clicking Just Stopped & Now You Can't Open? 113

Do This NOW (and DO NOT Do This)! 113

18
Why a Nightguard
Might NOT Work for You 118

A Strange Connection Between
Sleep & TMJ Problems *118*

19
No, You Probably Don't Need Braces
or All of Your Teeth Crowned 124

You Need an Accurate Diagnosis
and Conservative Treatment *124*

20
Being a Dental Instrument
For Mankind 128

21
Real Life Patient Stories.. 133

.... 140

Foreword
By Noah S. Siegel, MD

Marcie is a 33-year-old woman who came to see me with a chief complaint of recurrent ear infections. She explained to me that over the past couple years, she had frequent episodes of sharp ear pain which would radiate into her neck without symptoms of hearing loss or ear drainage. The pain would often wake her up at night and dramatically impact her day-to-day functioning. Furthermore, these episodes were frequently associated with severe headaches, neck pain and even ringing in her ear.

Many well-meaning physicians had treated her with antibiotics with variable success until they eventually sent her to an ear doctor (me) to sort things out.

Even though she had acute ear pain, Marcie was found to have completely normal ears, normal hearing testing, and an unremarkable exam of the head and neck. When I explained to Marcie that her ear examination was normal and that I suspected that her ear pain was attributable to her temporomandibular joint, it was difficult for her to believe. After all, she had been treated for ear infections for such a long time. How could this be? She had even been to her dentist who had taken an x-ray and told her, "Your pain is not dental." This made her even more incredulous since most people think that dentists have training in TMJ disorders (which sadly I have learned the vast majority do not).

Marcie's story is an extremely common one in the office of an otolaryngologist. We often see individuals for sinusitis/facial pain who have pristine sinuses. Patients often present to the emergency room, undergo extensive testing, are sent to an array of physicians including neurologists, allergists, and otolaryngologists and rarely get clear solutions to their problems.

One of the many things that I have learned over my 22 years of practicing otolaryngology is that finding a practitioner competent in managing TMJ problems is extremely difficult.

Most dentists are comfortable 'drilling and filling' and performing the dental interventions they learned in dental school. Beyond fashioning a simple 'night guard', most dentists shy away from managing temporomandibular joint problems.

In the interest of patient care, I really wish there were MANY more dentists like Dr. Patel who are willing to make the significant investment of time and money to take on the challenging patient population of individuals with TMJ disorders.

Noah S. Siegel, MD

Harvard Medical School
Director of Sleep Medicine and Sleep Surgery at Massachusetts Eye and Ear
Medical Director of Otolaryngology at Massachusetts Eye and Ear, Longwood

Introduction
By Jamison R. Spencer, DMD, MS

I look back on when I first started treating people with TMJ problems and realize now that much of what I was taught to do was wrong, or at the very least misguided.

I went right out of dental school in 1998 to take over a practice limited to the treatment of patients with TMJ disorders. That may not sound like a big deal, but at the time I was probably the first person to do so. You see, we don't get much education in dental school about TMJ problems. At my school I was the only one in my class to fit a patient with a simple nightguard, and that single case was the only practical experience I had.

We did have a few lectures on TMJ problems, and I distinctly remember a lecture that taught us how muscles can sometimes refer pain into your teeth, which seemed super complicated and very different from how tooth pain typically presents. As we walked out of the lecture I turned to my friend and said, "If I ever have a TMJ patient in my practice I'll refer them so fast it will make their head spin."

A few years after I said that I purchased a practice limited to seeing TMJ patients.

God definitely has a sense of humor.

My mentor had limited his practice to helping people with TMJ problems 8 years earlier and had a very good reputation in the Boise, Idaho area, which is where my wife and I are from. His overall paradigm (which he had developed over many years of studying with the top people in the field and implementing what he learned in his practice) was to treat with "splint therapy" and then when the patient got better he would modify how their teeth came together. Sometimes this modification of their bite was pretty simple and inexpensive and other times it required multiple teeth to be crowned, often costing the patient thousands of dollars, as well as requiring perfectly healthy teeth to be cut down during the crowning process. In this model the splint therapy was called "phase one" and the changing of the bite or occlusion was called "phase two." In my mentor's practice the vast majority of patients required phase two, either using crowns or moving the teeth through orthodontics.

This is how I practiced for the first couple of years as well, until one day I had a patient who had done fantastic with her splint therapy but said there was no way she could afford the phase two part of treatment. I called my mentor and asked him what to do. He said I should "wean the patient off her day splint." Problem was I didn't know how to do this—so he told me how, which involved the patient progressively wearing her day splint less and less, until she rarely wore it, but continuing to wear her nighttime appliance while she slept.

And it worked! She was able to "wean off" her day splint and her symptoms and dysfunction didn't come back!

I then had a bit of a moral dilemma. If I could wean people off of their day splints, why was I charging them thousands of dollars, and sometimes cutting down healthy teeth, to change their bite? This was a moral dilemma because fully half of my income was derived from performing these "phase two procedures."

I went and studied with Dr. Charles Holt of Fort Worth, Texas who had been successfully weaning patients off their day splints for years. I took the protocol that I learned from him and started to implement it in my practice and found similar success.

That year I announced to my dental colleagues that I would no longer be performing phase two treatments, but if the patient required such a bite change, I would work with their general dentist or orthodontist to help.

My practice doubled that year.

Dentists in my community liked that we were able to treat people so conservatively and with such good outcomes of relieving their pain and dysfunction.

That was over 20 years ago, and I've spent nearly that long teaching other dentists to provide the same type of conservative, predictable care that you'll read about in this book. TMJ problems can be extremely frustrating. We believe that the diagnosis, treatment and costs of treatment shouldn't contribute to that frustration.

In the early 2000's myself and a lot of other "TMJ dentists" started helping people with sleep apnea using oral appliances that our patients would wear while they slept. For several years I differentiated patients in my practice as "being there for TMJ" or "being there for sleep apnea."

Eventually we figured out that many of these people were suffering with both problems, and indeed in some of the people their sleep apnea was resulting in them having TMJ pain and dysfunction. Even though many of us have been doing this now for decades, the thought that sleep apnea, grinding the teeth (bruxism) and TMJ problems are often related is a very new concept for most medical and dental professionals, so don't be too surprised if you encounter dentists or doctors that haven't heard of all of the things you'll learn in the following pages.

This book is the result of the collaboration of multiple colleagues who have collectively helped tens of thousands of people suffering from TMJ related pain and dysfunction and represents their cumulative knowledge and experience of what actually works.

Since you are holding a copy of this book right now, I bet you are seeking care for yourself or a loved one. If you are, you've found the right place.

1
TMJ, The Great Imposter

Too often, people with chronic head pain are told by otherwise well-meaning and caring doctors that "It's all in your head" or "You'll have to learn to live with it—there's nothing you can do about it".

Unfortunately, migraine-like headaches, tension headaches, dizziness, ear pain, ear congestion, and eye, face, head, and neck pain are realities for sufferers. And yes, THEY are in your head!

THERE IS HOPE!

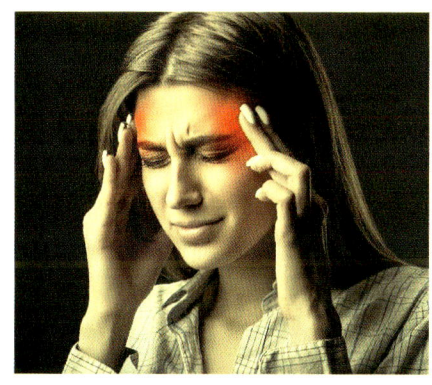

Often, there's a lot we can do about it. At least, there are many things that we can try before surgery!

Many times, a person wouldn't consider seeing a dentist for the above problems because their teeth are not painful. Or, at least the pain isn't perceived

13

as coming from the mouth. But that might not be the case.

We know that a person's mouth and teeth affect many aspects of one's overall health: for instance, when the bite is out of balance, the rest of the body can be out of whack. Did you know that many athletes wear bite orthotics, just like foot orthotics, to balance the bite? They find it increases strength and performance.

The symptoms of pain described earlier can often be related to the TMJ, muscle and/or jaw imbalances.

So, what is TMJ? Many people, doctors, nurses, and insurance companies use the term TMJ, but what is it?

TMJ is an abbreviation for "temporo-mandibular joint" or jaw joint. In fact, everybody has 2 TMJ's, one in front of each ear. The TM joint is formed by the temporal bone of the skull (temporo) and the lower jaw or mandible (mandibular).

The TMJ is the most complex joint in the entire body.

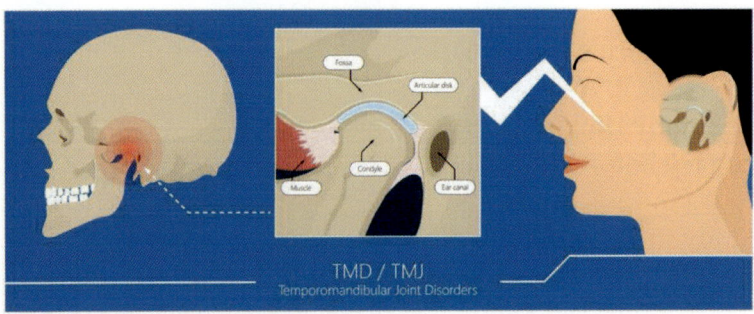

Your temporomandibular joints are gliding, sliding joints, unlike the ball and socket joints found elsewhere in your body. There is a fibrocartilage "disc" between the bones that allows the joint to glide and slide smoothly.

It is the only joint in the body where the end point in the range of motion is not defined by muscles, ligaments and tendons but instead by how the teeth come together. If the bite is NOT right, the joint is pulled out of alignment and serious problems can develop.
And, if you lose your teeth, or they shift a lot, forget about it! The jaw won't even know where to go!

These TM joints move every time we talk, chew, or swallow (and we swallow around 2000 times a day!). In a normal swallow your upper and lower teeth come together. Doing this more than 2000 times a day with an unstable bite causes the surrounding muscles to work extra hard. This starts a cycle of tissue damage, muscle tenderness, and pain.

Pain is the end result—a symptom. It is not the cause. Pain is your body's way of informing you of a problem, a defense mechanism. In this case, the problem is an imbalance in your jaw.

This is really important to understand. If PAIN were the real culprit, then taking pain relievers would be the solution. But since the real issue is the IMBALANCE, taking pain relievers only covers up the problem and never resolves the cause.

The result can be dependence on pain medication or systems that are called by the medical community, PAIN MANAGEMENT. When we help you get to the CAUSE of the problem, we can minimize the use of medications or pain management systems.

TMJ problems often start innocently...maybe with something as little as the muscles not moving in harmony on both sides. Loud clicking and popping sounds in the ear are NOT normal, with or without pain. The sound is an indication that your gliding, sliding disc is displaced forward, out of place—dislocated!

If your knee made crunching noises every time you walked, would you be worried? You might not be able to walk properly.

Well, what about a clicking jaw? This could eventually affect your ability to chew, swallow, and talk—things we often take for granted. Why wait until you can't chew, swallow or talk? Being proactive and finding the cause early could save a lot of pain and money down the road.

TMJ disease may progress from muscle soreness and tenderness to clicking and popping with any jaw movement, to locking when the mouth is closed or open, to limited opening, and finally to total breakdown of the jaw bone. As the stages progress, pain usually increases. In the early stages, surprisingly, there might NOT be any pain and the damage goes on silently. Remember, as we said before, pain is our body's way of telling us there's something wrong—we would do well to listen when it speaks!

Some of the symptoms of TMD (temporomandibular disorder) are:
- TMJ pain
- Headaches
- Neck pain
- Limited neck rotation

- Ear pain
- Ear congestion
- Limited mouth opening
- Pain spreading to the eyes, shoulder, neck, or back
- Clicking or popping of the jaw
- Locking jaw
- Clenching and grinding of the teeth
- Dizziness
- Teeth pain or sensitivity without any cavities or oral health disease
- Gums receding
- Broken fillings, teeth and caps (crowns)
- Trigeminal neuralgia.

The main nerve controlling the TMJ is the trigeminal nerve. The trigeminal nerve supplies input to the teeth, the jaws, sinuses, the opening/closing muscles, the chewing muscles, and are coupled to the Atlas and Axis (C1 + C2) vertebrae in the neck.

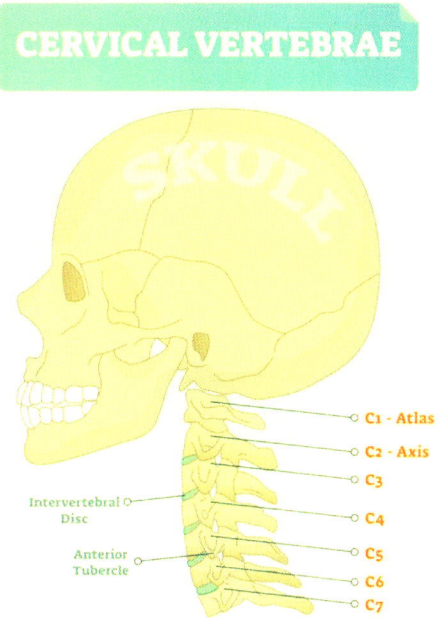

There are 10 cranial nerves that originate in the brain and control our bodily functions. There are 2 nerves, the trigeminal and facial, that affect the 136 different muscles or 68 pairs of "dental muscles". Of all the cranial nerves in the brain, the trigeminal provides MORE THAN 50% OF ALL THE INPUT INTO THE BRAIN.

With so much brain input, you can appreciate how an issue with your TMJ (triggering the trigeminal nerves in an abnormal way) can lead to problems in the rest of your nervous system and may not only cause abnormal muscles contractions but also impact other brain/nerve-controlled functions as well.

When your lower jaw moves downward (opening your mouth), it generates a pulling force, loosening the muscle in your neck around C2 or the axis vertebrae. Likewise, the jaw moving upward (closing your mouth) generates a pressure which tightens muscles in the neck around your C2 vertebrae. This means that when your bite is off and has lost its height, it could aggravate the muscles around C2 in your neck when your mouth is closed.

So, a problem with your TMJ could affect the position of your C2, neck pain, and possible collapse of your neck vertebrae. And with a domino effect, the C2/axis plays a key role in the balance of the entire spine.

And the problem works both ways. When there is a posture problem and/or the spine is too curved, it could affect how the jaw lies because of the interaction of the muscles that connect the jaw to the rest of the body.

That's why an examination to evaluate a potential TMJ problem may also include an analysis of your posture (which could be a formal test or an experienced professional just observing your posture). Sometimes, a postural problem can, by nature of the interactions of the muscles contribute to a jaw imbalance as well. Such a jaw imbalance might result in grinding or clenching, symptoms, which might show up long before any pain.

Have you have been told you grind or clench your teeth? Do you have some of these signs of grinding or clenching?

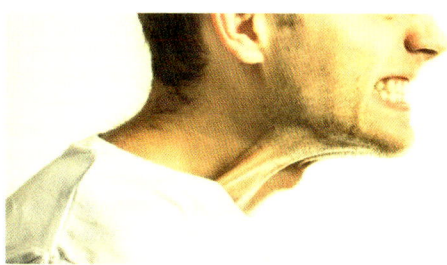

- Worn down or chipped teeth
- Recession of the gums (without gum disease)
- Notches in the teeth
- Indentations on the sides of the teeth
- A taller or shorter looking tooth or multiple teeth
- Extra bone growth (called tori), on the roof of the mouth, sides of the upper or lower jaw, or inside of the lower jaw (the bumps you might feel with your tongue)
- Broken caps (crowns) and/or fillings
- Teeth that are sensitive to cold

So, what is the connection between these factors?

Clenching or grinding your teeth might indicate that there's an imbalance. It also might point to one of many other different causes (preview of coming attractions in chapters 6, 7 & 8).

Many studies have found that people with TMJ issues also have sleep breathing issues. During sleep, when the airway (the breathing tube in your throat) collapses, the body's automatic response is to open it up. The brain will do anything to get oxygen! One of the things it may do is force the muscles to push the lower jaw forward in order to open the airway and allow for breathing. Another way your brain may try to open your airway is by causing you to clench your teeth to keep that little tube from collapsing back on itself.

Whichever path your brain chooses, it is beyond your conscious control. This is one of the reasons some people who swear they never clench or grind have heavy wear patterns on their teeth (which typically take years to develop). It's their brain's way of protecting them from suffocating and it's triggered by a lack of oxygen in the bloodstream. Your brain is willing to sacrifice your teeth to get oxygen.

Some of the consequences of sleep breathing disorders are cardiovascular issues, high blood pressure, strokes, daytime sleepiness, snoring, atrial fibrillation, depression, and short-term memory loss. (More on this important sleep apnea/TMJ connection in Chapter 18.)

TMD is commonly linked to chronic fatigue syndrome, fibromyalgia, and sleep breathing disorders. In fact, the NHLBI or National Heart, Lung and Blood Institute considers sleep apnea (sleep breathing disorder) to be a TMJ disorder.

You might hear different terms for problems involving the TMJ. Dentists sometimes refer to it as TMD (the D standing for dysfunction). Some may call it neuralgia (nerve problem), others myalgia (muscle problem) and yet others, arthralgia (joint problem). Whatever it's called, getting to the ROOT CAUSE of the problem is the best way to manage it and prevent it from getting worse.

And, if an airway blockage at night is the cause, then resolving the airway issue will be the first step in helping to relieve the TMJ symptoms so you can get a more restful and refreshing night's sleep.

But remember, you probably only sleep 7-8 hours a night. What happens during your waking hours is just as important. So, in this book we will discuss the many other factors that can play a role in continued discomfort, even after the sleep issue is resolved.

Being evaluated by someone who appreciates the entirety of the airway-posture-joint-muscle-nerve-teeth complex is the best way to assure that YOU will get a resolution to any discomfort you might be experiencing.

2
It's Not All in Your Head

*Even Though It's Not All in Your Head,
What IS in Your Head
Can Make a Huge Difference!*

Chanel was the life of the party. She was clever and quick witted and ready to lead the masses onto life's dance floor.

When the facial pain wouldn't stop though, she found it harder to dance through life. The movement made her nauseous and the loud music came at her like a freight train. Her meals went from carefully planned and prepared to whichever fast-food joint had the softest food and the shortest line. Chanel was in bed for hours, but sleep was now fragmented with bouts of pain and worry about how she would function the next morning. Pain was the reason she got up in the morning, and the reason she crawled back into bed at the end of the day.

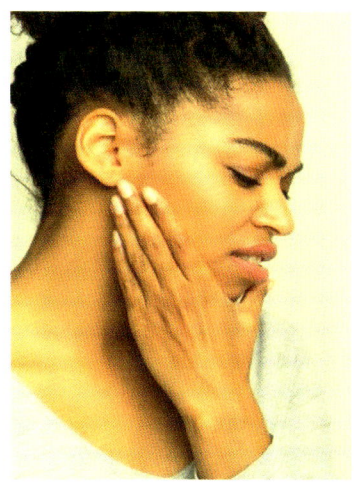
What do we do when our pain seems to take over our entire existence? What do we do when the doctor tells us the pain is "all in our head"?

Well, it IS... your pain IS all IN YOUR HEAD! The pain you feel is a very real message sent from your injured body part back to your brain. What you DO with that message is up to YOU!

In this book we will discuss the possible causes and treatments of the pain and other symptoms you are feeling. But before we get into that, let's set a foundation of how powerful your mind is and how you can use it to fuel the recovery and heal the causes of your symptoms. Afterall, what you 'feed your mind' WILL affect how you manage pain and recovery. And we're here to help!!

A very important tool in your doctor's healing toolbox is a whole subsection of psychology, called pain psychology.

A pain psychologist specializes in addressing the mind-body connection by walking you through cognitive behavioral therapy like grounding, mindfulness, and radical acceptance. They also evaluate you for underlying depression and anxiety which are important considerations (50% of chronic pain patients are struggling with this as well—a possible connection we will discuss in chapter 18).

Because neurologists have found VERY powerful connections between what we say to ourselves and what we feel, addressing any depression and anxiety in concert with the pain will help the success of overall improvement.

So how can YOU use your most powerful tool, your mind, to your healing advantage? Pain psychologists have found the following 4 principles are a great place to start:

1. **Self-Monitoring:** We spend a lot of time distracting ourselves from our pain. To truly self-monitor you need to open yourself up and look straight down the barrel of your pain again. Look for patterns in your pain... what activities or circumstances in your environment come right before your pain escalates? Write these down. Recognizing this list will give you ownership over their power. Pain psychologists can then help you develop a plan to reduce or restructure your environment to minimize these triggers.

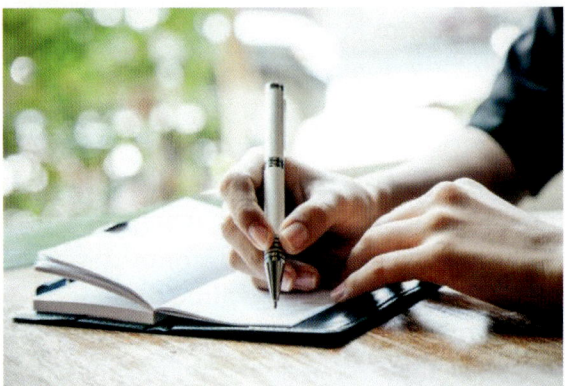

2. **Relaxation:** When we experience chronic pain, our body switches into and out of a state of fight or flight to protect us. If this happens daily, we

quickly default to 'fight or flight' the next time we encounter even the smallest pain or distress... putting us into a more delicate psychological state. Physical relaxation, like progressive muscle relaxation, will turn down the volume on our fight or flight reaction to pain which makes the pain 'feel' less and puts us in a better headspace to deal with any future distress.

3. **Thinking differently about your symptoms:** Research has shown that catastrophizing, or thinking the worst, leads to an increased pain perception. Using self-statements that are positive like, "My pain may be worse today, but tomorrow will be better" actually creates physical changes in the nervous system that can help alter how much pain you 'feel.'

4. **Behavioral strategies:** Pace your activities... don't go out and eat a bag of beef jerky once you start to feel better. Be more assertive to get the help you need from those around you. Recognizing your triggers and eliminating them may require the help of your friends and family.

If pain has become a part of your personality, these tools give you permission to let that part of your past go and create a new YOU. If you have an injured joint, your new YOU may always have times of discomfort, but your newfound ability to identify and treat yourself during flare-ups will help keep pain from encompassing all of you... pain will just be a little freckle on your NEW YOU.

This mind-body connection is a powerful tool and could be a key to your success and progression on your healing journey.

3

"I've Got TMJ!"

The Most Amazing Joint in the Body!

Why is the temporomandibular joint, or TMJ, the most intricate joint in the body? Well, that tiny little space is packed full of complicated anatomy functioning in harmony with the same joint on the other side of your head! If your jaw joints aren't working well together it's way harder to eat, speak or even breathe properly.

The TMJ is also the only joint whose movement has a rigid endpoint of closure—which is dictated by the teeth.

This chapter will focus on the bones of the head that make up the solid components of the TMJ, as well as the key cartilage structure that allows this joint to function.

Once the intricacies of the TMJ are understood, it becomes easier to comprehend how pain and dysfunction can occur.

Bones of the temporomandibular joint

The TMJ is categorized as a complex joint, even though it only has 2 bones—not 3 as do most complex joints. The third component that classifies this joint as complex is the little fibrocartilage disc that glides between your mandible and your skull.

The section of the skull that forms the upper part of the TMJ is called the temporal bone. The parts of the temporal bone that work with the TMJ are a little pocket called the **glenoid fossa** and a downward slope called the **articular eminence**. And then of course the jaw bone or mandible has a little ball on the end that fits in that spot called the **condylar head**, or condyle. The condylar head of the mandible provides the hinge motion when you open your mouth.

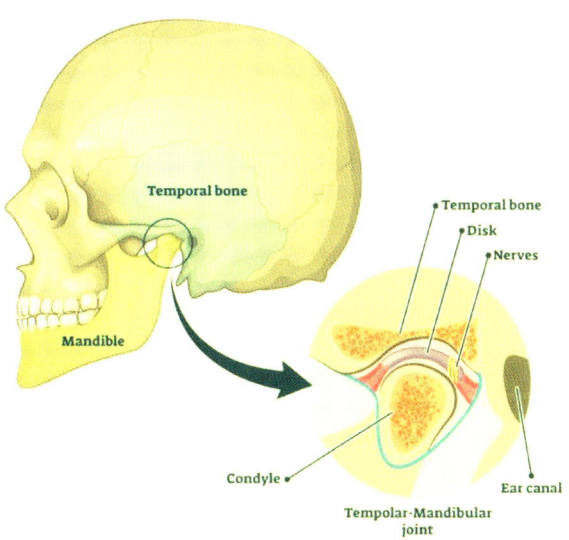

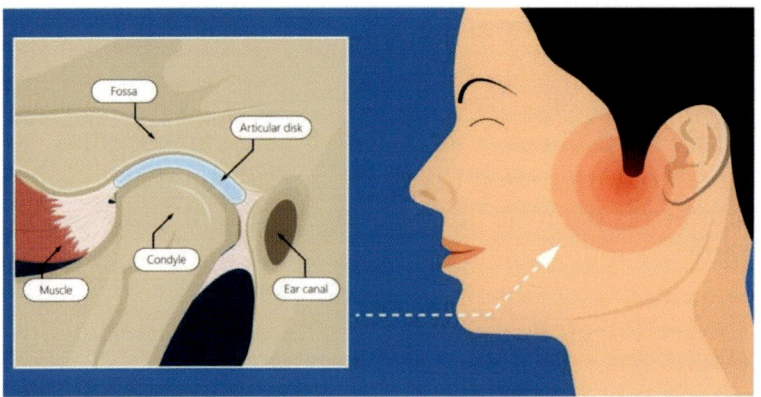

Now that you know all the "hard" facts about the bone, let's talk cartilage. Between all these bones there is a little disc called the **articular or articulating disc**. This disc is a special kind of cartilage that moves with the mandible to provide a cushion between the condyle of the mandible and the temporal bone.

It is this disc that makes the magic happen, allowing each of us to talk and sing and eat and laugh and yodel if we want to.

The disc is made of fibrocartilage which is different from the cartilage in most other joints. Fibrocartilage gives the disc strength, makes it less susceptible to aging, and allows it to repair on its own.

The widest portion of the disc sits behind the condyle and right in front of the ear. The thinnest portion is the middle, and it gets wider again as it goes over the condyle. Picture an hourglass on its side and you've got the right shape of a healthy disc.

If the structure of the mandibular fossa and/or the condyle change due to injury or wear and tear, the shape of the disc will also change. As you will read further in the book, this can lead to changes in how the joint functions.

In addition, the disc does not have any nerves, so it doesn't feel pain.

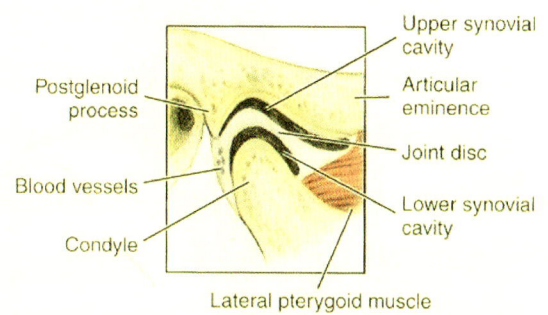

The placement of the articulating disc produces two spaces within the joint. The space above the disc and below the temporal bone's mandibular fossa is referred to as the superior compartment or **upper synovial cavity**. The space below the disc and above the condyle of the mandible is called the inferior compartment or **lower synovial cavity**. Those are big names for such little spaces!

Each of those spaces are filled with an egg-white-like fluid called **synovial fluid**. This fluid provides nutrients and lubrication to the joint and classifies the TMJ as a synovial joint.

The upper or superior space allows you to move your lower jaw forward, backward and sideways. The lower or inferior compartment is responsible for the opening/closing (or lowering and raising) movement of your jaw.

The most stable position of the TM joint is when your lips are together, your teeth are apart, and the tongue is lightly touching the roof of the mouth.

This photo shows the condyle of the mandible in a forward position, where it sits when the mouth is open

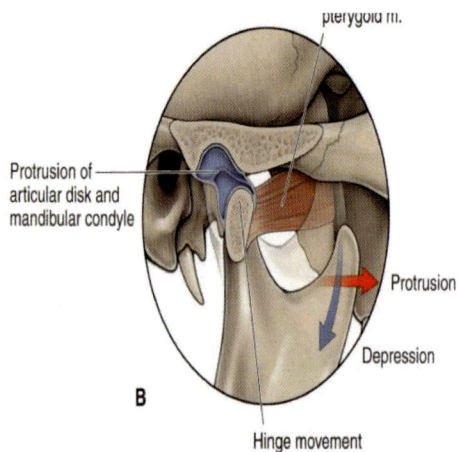

The tissue behind the disc is referred to as the **retrodiscal tissue**. The job of this tissue is to prevent the disc from becoming dislocated in front of the condyle or said another way, to keep it from rotating too far over the condyle.

The middle portion of this retrodiscal tissue houses a LOT of blood vessels and nerves. As the lower jaw moves forward, this area fills with blood. Unlike the disc, this tissue is sensitive to pain and inflammation.

Behind the retrodiscal tissue is where the **external ear canal** is located. The ear canal is so close to the TMJ that it slightly changes shape as your mouth opens and closes during daily functions such as smiling, chewing and talking.

This very close proximity to the TMJ is why injury or inflammation to the joint can cause symptoms such as ear pain, congestion and/or ringing in the ear. Oftentimes people will seek care from an ear, nose and throat doctor because they are having ear pain—not knowing the cause of their pain is not the ear but is actually the temporomandibular joint.

This is a simple overview of the bone and articulating disc that make up the TMJ. It is the complex movement capability of this joint, forward, backward, up, down, and side to side, that allows us to nourish our bodies, communicate with others, and breathe properly.

In other words—it's a pretty important joint! (Unless you don't care about eating, speaking or breathing…)

4

Chewing is Awesome! (When It Doesn't Hurt)

The Muscles of Mastication & How We Chew

Now that we have discussed the temporomandibular joint let's talk about the soft tissue components—muscles, tendons, and ligaments. *Without those, the joint would not be very useful!*

There are 3 groups of muscles in the human body. The first two groups, **smooth muscles,** and **cardiac muscles** are found in the heart, intestines, gallbladder, urinary bladder, blood vessels, and other internal organs. They are called involuntary muscles because we have no conscious control

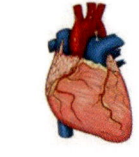
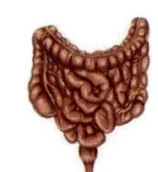
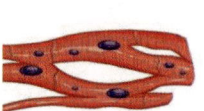
Cardiac muscle
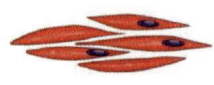
Smooth muscle

over them. (It's kind of nice to have all those body parts on autopilot!).

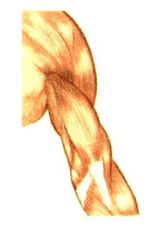

Skeletal muscles are the ones that move our body, provide stability, and give it shape. Each muscle is made of many elastic fibers. These muscles make up 40 to 50% of human body weight (think biceps, quads, 6 pack abs, etc.).

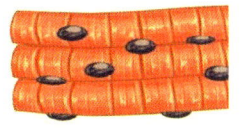
Skeletal muscle

Skeletal muscles can also generate heat (that's why you shiver in the cold).

There are approximately 650 skeletal muscles in the human body and our minds have voluntary control over all of them.

Skeletal muscles are attached to the bones (or sometimes other muscles or tissues) at two or more places by **tendons**. The **muscle origin** is the place where the tendon attaches the muscle to the bone that doesn't move when the muscle contracts. Attachment to the bone that moves during the contraction is called the **muscle insertion**.

Skeletal muscles can only create movement by shortening and pulling the part it inserts to against the

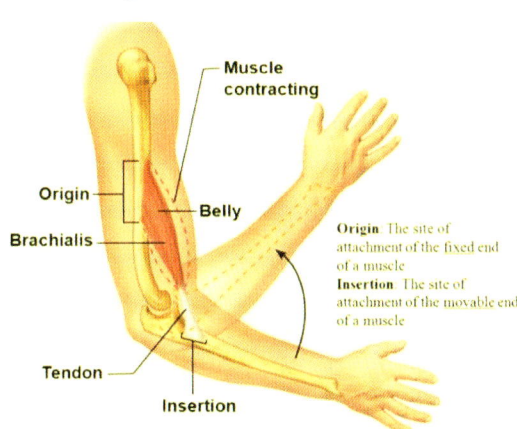

part it originates from, therefore moving body parts in relation to each other.

Most muscles work in antagonistic (or opposite) pairs. For example, jaw opening muscles work together with jaw-closing muscles. Muscles that extend the arm work together with muscles that flex the arm. We will talk more about that later in this chapter.

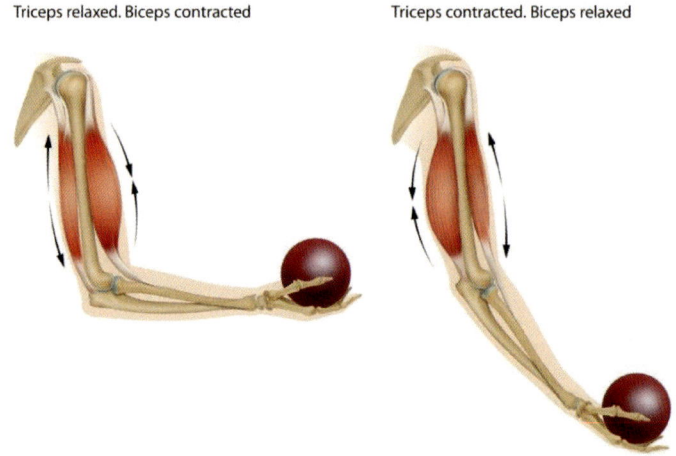

Skeletal muscles are made up of "motor units." These tiny units are made of neuron and muscle fibers. The size and type of the motor unit determines how resilient and fast the muscle is.

There are many muscles in the head and neck that create the incredibly fine-tuned symphony of movements allowing speech, chewing, swallowing, breathing, maintaining posture, facial expression, etc. (Think about having dinner with your friends and talking, laughing, eating, drinking, and breathing all at the same time!) And it's all accomplished by shortening and then relaxing the individual muscle fibers.

Bones, muscles, tendons, and ligaments are all part of the musculoskeletal system. Before we dive into a discussion about specific jaw muscles, let's talk about tendons and ligaments. (The support staff without which the body would not function! Also, it is often injury or inflammation of ligaments or tendons that produces the most painful symptoms. We will discuss those in more detail in a later chapter.)

Both ligaments and tendons are made of dense fibrous connective tissue, but they have different functions.

Tendons and ligaments do not have a robust blood supply. Since the body heals by transporting all the necessary healing nutrients and building blocks inside the blood, once tendons or ligaments are injured, the healing can be difficult and can take a long time.

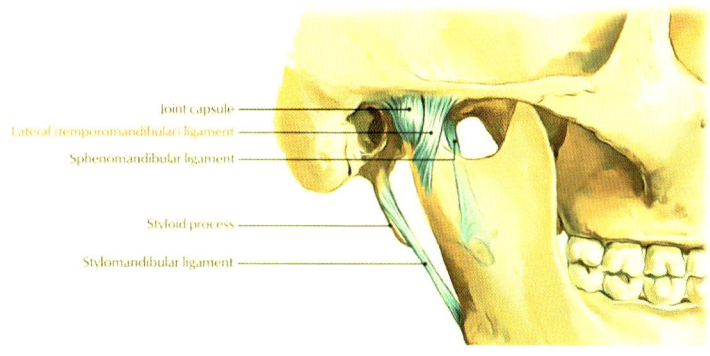

Ligaments attach bone to bone and protect the joints by providing boundaries for joint mobility. The more movable the joint is the more it relies on ligaments for stability. Excessive stretching causes **ligament sprain** (anyone who ever rolled their ankle can relate). People who are hyper-mobile ("double-jointed") have loose ligaments and can injure the joints easily because the "ligament ropes" are not strong enough to protect the joints from overextension.

The TMJ is a very mobile and complex joint and has several ligaments associated with it. As we discussed in the previous chapter, the cartilage disc inside the TMJ is held in place by two ligaments. The joint capsule that surrounds the TMJ is also made of ligaments. There are two other ligaments outside the joint that connect the skull to the mandible and guard against overextension of the joint.

Tendons attach muscles to bones and facilitate movement. Tendons are very strong—the strongest soft tissue in the body. Even so, they can become injured when the muscle is overused, causing **strain and inflammation.** This condition is called **tendinitis** (tennis elbow is an example of tendinitis).

Now let's talk muscles. The muscles that move the lower jaw are collectively called the **muscles of mastication** (chewing muscles). There are primary and secondary muscles of mastication.

Primary Muscles of Mastication (Chewing)

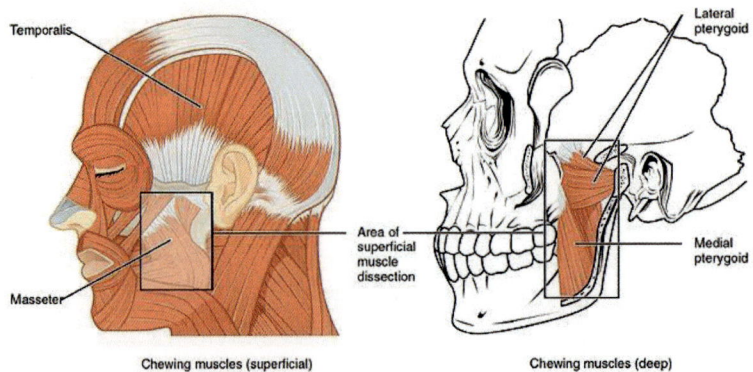

There are 4 primary muscles of mastication: **masseter, temporalis, medial pterygoid, and lateral pterygoid.** These muscles originate at different points of the skull and insert into the lower jaw since this is the only bone in your head that you can move.

Let's discuss each of these 4 muscles to help us understand the role they could play in TMJ dysfunction.

The masseter is the most noticeable jaw muscle. They are the muscles that define the shape of your face along your jaw line. It is the strongest muscle in the body by weight. It provides a very powerful chewing stroke and allows the back teeth to close with a force of up to 200 pounds. (Anyone who ever bit their tongue will attest to the strength of this muscle—ouch!) This muscle is very active during teeth clenching.

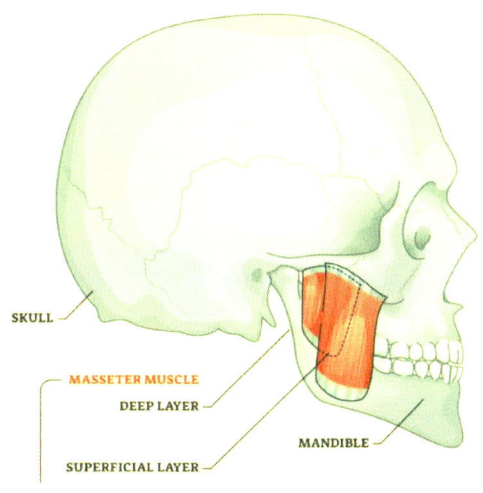

TEMPORALIS

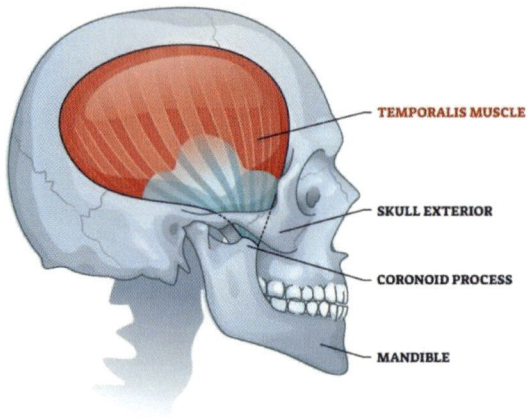

The **temporalis** is a large fan-shaped muscle that is located on the side of the skull. It attaches to the lower jaw by a large temporal tendon (the white areas in the picture above are the tendons). Overuse of this muscle and strain of the temporal tendon can often be a source of headaches and can even mimic migraines. We will talk about that more in future chapters as well.

Because its often the source of the headache, some people call the temporalis a "headache muscle". But the name actually comes from the Latin word "tempus" meaning "time". The temporalis muscle covers the temporal bone and the hair over this bone is often the first hair to turn gray.

Working together both right and left temporal muscles function to close the jaw, stabilize the jaw, and move it back. If only one side is activated, it will move the jaw to the same side. This is also considered a posture muscle because it helps to maintain the position of the lower jaw at rest. As you can

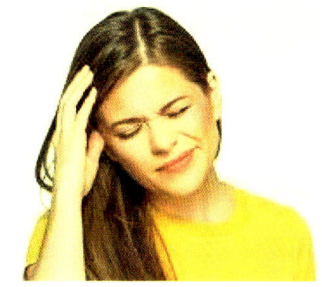

imagine, the temporal muscles are very active during clenching.

MEDIAL PTERYGOID

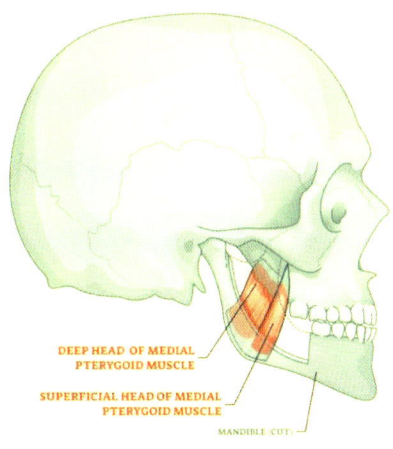

The **medial pterygoid** is a muscle that forms a sling together with the masseter muscle to support the lower jaw. Because it is located on the inside of the mandible it is hard to access. However, if you have ever had an injection to numb a lower back tooth or molar (way in the back of your mouth) that injection was placed next to your medial pterygoid.

LATERAL PTERYGOID

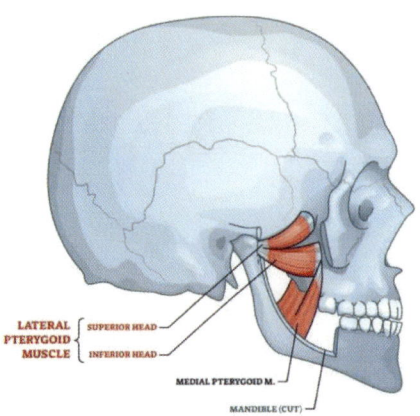

The **lateral pterygoid** is located really far up and towards the back, and is virtually impossible to touch. It is divided into two portions and is the only muscle of mastication that facilitates jaw opening.

Secondary Muscles of Mastication (Chewing)

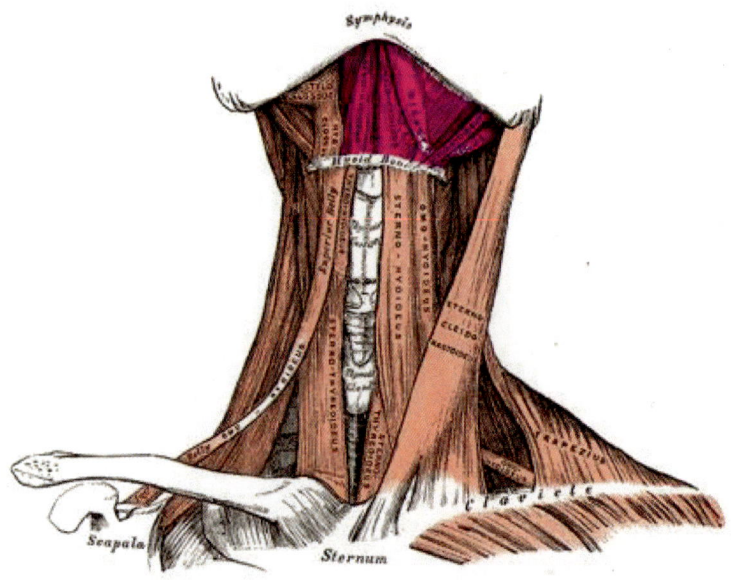

Secondary muscles of mastication assist in chewing but are mostly in charge of swallowing. They are located on the front of the neck. These muscles attach to a small hyoid bone located under the lower jaw. They are divided into 4 pairs of supra hyoid muscles (above the hyoid bone) and 4 pairs of infra hyoid muscles (below the hyoid bone). Some of them, together with the lateral pterygoid muscle, assist in opening the lower jaw. The **Buccinator** (the cheek muscle) is also considered to be a secondary muscle of mastication.

The Tongue

The **tongue** is a collection of several muscles that participate in the process of chewing by forming the food and moving it around your mouth. The tongue itself is made up of 4 groups of muscles and there are also 4 muscles that attach it to the lower jaw, the hyoid bone, and the skull.

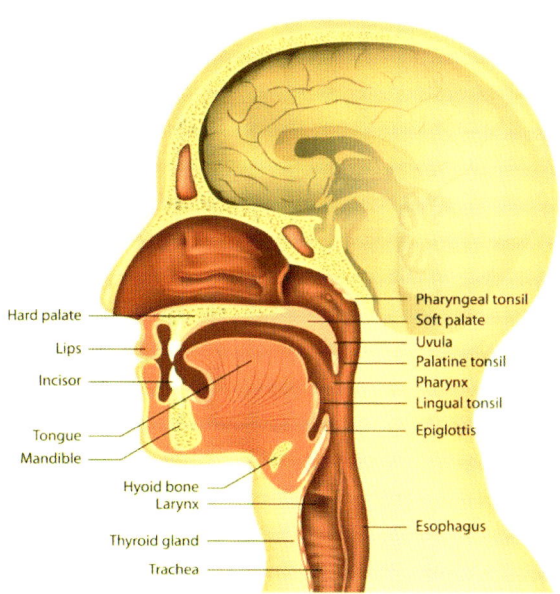

The simple process of chewing (something that we do without giving it too much thought), involves the precise coordination of more than 20 pairs of different muscles all working in harmony by contracting and relaxing in a very specific manner that we don't have to think about.

When everything is functioning well, it is a beautiful, smooth, orchestra-like movement. When it's not functioning well, the complexity of the system requires a thorough understanding of all the intricate details to analyze what might be amiss.

The complex anatomy of this area is just one of the reasons it's so important to work with a professional who has a great deal of experience and training dealing with TMJ dysfunction.

5
Lips Together, Teeth Apart

*The Best Way to Avoid & Treat
Many TMJ Problems
(Easier Said Than Done)*

You could make one very simple change in your behavior and feel better.

This change doesn't require eating anything healthy, taking a pill or wearing a brace. You won't even have to work up a sweat. If you could just do this ONE THING, it might help relieve your pain.

What is this magical fix?

It's so simple, it sounds too good to be true—always keep your teeth slightly apart, except when you are swallowing.

That's right! Your teeth should only touch for a fraction of a second when you swallow. Even when you are eating, your teeth don't exactly touch much—there is food in between!

While this is SIMPLE, it might not be so easy. Habits, as we all know, are hard to break.

The reason this is such a "revolutionary" thought is because of time—time under pressure, to be more precise. Ideally our teeth should only touch for about 10-15 minutes per day. That is about 1% of the day. Pretty easy to understand how a significant deviation from this "norm" can cause problems like jaw joint pain, jaw muscle pain and/or clicking and popping in the jaw joints!

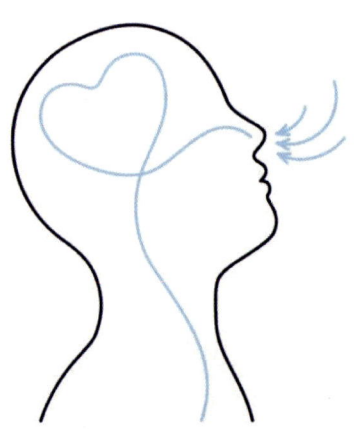

Breathing through the nose

This oral posture—lips lightly together, tongue passively on the roof of the mouth, teeth slightly separated—sets the stage for NASAL breathing. Nasal breathing is ideal as the nose does the very important job of filtering, disinfecting, warming, and moisturizing the air we breathe in before it gets to the throat and lungs.

Where should your lips be?

The lips should be lightly together, passive, and relaxed. At rest. There should be no need to force them together. There should be no tension or muscle contraction. The lips may be slightly apart, but this wouldn't necessarily mean the person is breathing through the mouth. Why? Because it depends on the position of the tongue.

Where should the tongue be?

All this talk about where the teeth should be begs the question of "where should my tongue go?" Well, the tip of the tongue should be lightly resting against the roof of the mouth, just behind the front teeth. Think of this position as if you were about to say "no". Depending on the size of your tongue relative to the shape of your lower teeth, the back part of your tongue may be resting slightly on the inside chewing surfaces of your back teeth (molars). If you were to get an upper-cut to the jaw, you would likely bite your tongue.

Why is it so important for teeth to only touch when swallowing?

Ultimately it comes down to the amount of TIME UNDER PRESSURE and the laws of physics. Spending too much time with your teeth touching for a few weeks or even a month will likely cause very few problems. However, as TIME UNDER PRESSURE increases, problems are more likely to occur.

There are several structures that could be affected. Overworked muscles can cause pain in your face and in your teeth. Pain can even radiate up into your eye, into your sinus area, into your jaw bones and into your ears.

Pressure over time can cause the disc inside your jaw joint to dislocate. Oftentimes people will hear or feel a click or a pop in their jaw joint when they open and close. That is the joint relocating (going back into place) when you open and dislocating when you close. This frequent dislocation can lead to your jaw locking and can also be quite painful.

The teeth can also sustain fractures over time. If this has happened to you, you know that fractured teeth can be very painful and costly to repair. Sometimes fractures are not fixable, necessitating the removal of the tooth.

Could a daytime orthotic help?

Sometimes a trained dentist might send you home with a temporary device that can help with clenching and also remind you to rest their jaw. It's a simple little device that can be thought of as two lakes connected by a river. It has 2 pads, one on each end, filled with a little water (the lakes) which sit between the upper and lower molars (back teeth). The pads are connected by a thin tube of water that wraps around the front teeth (the river).

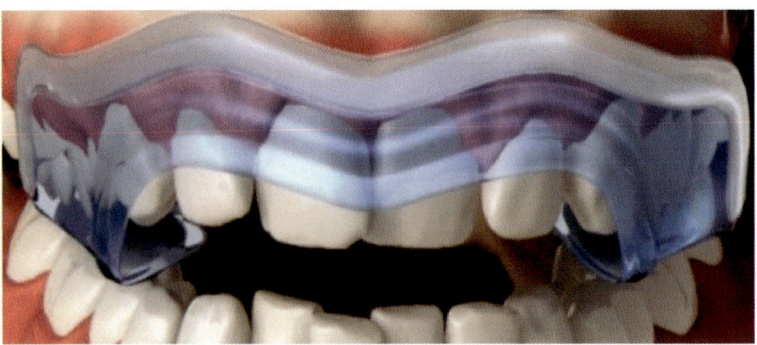

This device can be worn for a few days (up to a week or so). It's passive too, meaning that it's not meant to be bitten or chewed on. Upon pressure, the water will move from one side of the jaw to the other until it is balanced.

This often helps you realize, and your doctor diagnose that you are clenching. By balancing the pressure, it helps the muscles relax. Then when the muscles have a chance to relax, you may need to transition to a solid, more long-term, and durable orthotic that maintains the balanced position. These are designed to be worn for a longer time, typically until pain symptoms subside.

If so, will I have to wear the orthotic all the time, forever?

The objective of wearing a daytime orthotic, whether it is a temporary one or one made of a more durable material, is to reduce or eliminate pain and reduce or eliminate clicking or popping in the jaw joint(s). A daytime orthotic is essentially a bio-feedback device, meant to reduce or eliminate self-destructive daytime habits. Once those goals are achieved, the process of weaning off the daytime orthotic begins. The ultimate goal is that a daytime orthotic is NOT a forever appliance.

What effects can come from proper positioning?

When there is harmony between the position of your tongue, teeth, and lips, good things happen. There is less pressure on the tissues inside your jaw joint and there is less contraction of the muscles associated with your jaw. Commonly, this will result in more jaw joint comfort, and a more comfortable feeling in your jaw muscles since they will not be so overworked.

Often, there will be substantial healing within your jaw joint itself because the disc is then allowed to remain in a more comfortable, stable and physiologic position.

It's the perfect anatomic example of less resulting in more.

6

Yes, Stress Can Cause Clenching & Grinding, But So Can…

Medications and Other Things that Contribute to Clenching & Grinding

Medical science still doesn't fully understand all the causes of **bruxism** (the clenching and grinding of your teeth), and it's one of the main contributors to temporomandibular disorders (TMD).

In fact, bruxism may be a combination of many things, including genetic, physical, and psychological factors. We do know that bruxism has been a documented part of the human condition for thousands of years; for example, even the Bible mentions the "gnashing of teeth" (although it was then attributed to sin, and to those unfortunates eternally damned to hell).

There are some medical conditions that seem to predispose a person to bruxism including: Parkinson's Disease, dementia, and epilepsy.

Recent research has also shown that some bruxism may be related to sleep conditions including sleep apnea, as mentioned in chapter one. So, if you clench AND snore or have other sleep problems, consider completing a sleep study to determine if there is an underlying sleep-related root cause of your bruxism. It is often "good news" if someone with TMD also has sleep apnea, since we can commonly manage both conditions with one dental device (or with CPAP and a "nightguard" if bruxism persists with sleep apnea resolution). We'll go into this possible connection more in depth in chapter 18.

OSA/bruxism

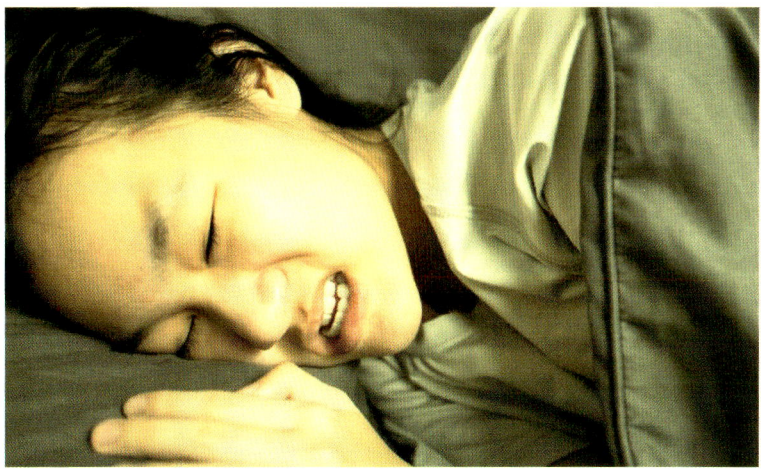

We know that many people who don't have sleep apnea may clench or grind their teeth when sleeping. While emotional stress may not be the root cause of this type of bruxism, it does tend to increase the FORCE and FREQUENCY of clenching or grinding events. This is one reason why so many experience more jaw, neck, and headache pain during stressful periods.

Daytime clenching may also occur and could be related to stress, or it may just be a learned coping habit that needs to be broken.

Besides stress and sleep apnea, what else can cause bruxism? Would you be surprised to learn that one answer may be in your medicine cabinet?

Here's how...

Many people who are dealing with stress also experience increased pain and anxiety. Pain management physicians are well aware of the relationship between pain and mood disorders, such as anxiety and/or depression. It seems that those who have pain are at higher risk for mood disorders, and vice versa, because jaw pain symptoms may be a physical manifestation of certain mood disorders.

It can be challenging to understand which came first, but research suggests those with anxiety tend to experience more muscle pain, while depression was more closely linked to jaw joint pain. (Journal of Pain, 1/16/2013)

Many dentists and physicians are taught in school that "all TMJ patients are crazy," and that their TMJ patients are just NUTS. But this is untrue! Unless you understand that NUTS is an acronym meaning "Not Understanding Their Symptoms." It may be the doctors themselves who are "NUTS," because they received so little training about the TM joint in medical or dental school, and don't really understand what's going on.

A common way to manage mood disorders is via prescription of an anti-anxiety or anti-depression medication. It is ironic and unfortunate that some of these medications, specifically those called SSRI's and SNRI's, have side effects that include jaw clenching or grinding, and increased jaw pain or other TMD-related symptoms such as headaches.

Perhaps more concerning is that some medical providers seem unaware of this connection, or at least they're unaware of the possibility that bruxism and its debilitating consequences can be caused by the very drugs they are prescribing.

So, what are these medications that are linked to bruxism, and in turn potentially cause (or worsen) the symptoms associated with TMD?

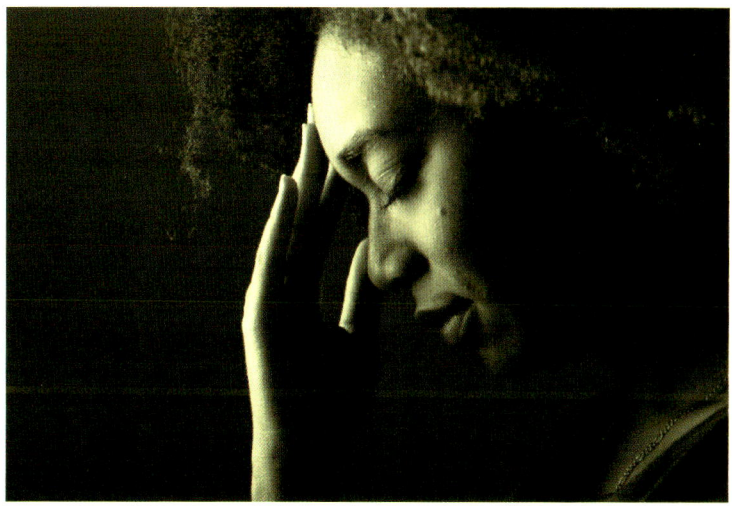

Research has shown that they are **serotonin-norepinephrine reuptake inhibitors (SNRIs)** that treat, among others, the following common mood disorders:

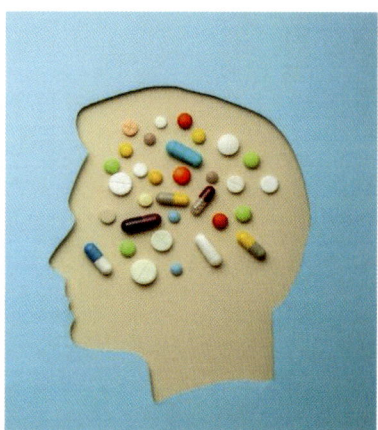

- Anxiety or depression
- Post-partum depression
- Bipolar disorder
- OCD
- Psychotic conditions
- Panic disorder
- Social anxiety disorder / social phobia
- Bulimia
- Hot flashes
- And interestingly: fibromyalgia, chronic pain (low back, joint, muscle), nerve pain

Common SNRIs:
- Prozac (Fluoxetine)
- Zoloft (Sertraline)
- Paxil (Paroxetine)
- Celexa (Citalopram)
- Lexapro (Escitalopram)
- Effexor (Venlafaxine)
- Pristiq (Desvenlafaxine)
- Cymbalta (Duloxetine)

For the technically minded, these drugs work by preventing reuptake of the *neurotransmitters* serotonin or norepinephrine (substances the brain uses to send messages from one nerve cell to another) at the synapse, or the space between the nerve cells. This means these chemicals remain for a longer time in the synapse.

Medicine doesn't fully understand what causes mood disorders such as depression, but they appear to be related to some combination of chemical imbalances in the brain, or a deficiency of serotonin. And while we also don't understand precisely how these medications work, clinical trials have substantiated that these drugs tend to be beneficial for the mood disorders for which they are typically prescribed.

Everyone responds to medications differently—while some may experience few (if any) side effects, others certainly do. Just think of some of the crazy side effects listed on drug TV commercials! It may take a few weeks of use for these symptoms to develop, and while many people do not experience an increase in bruxism, headache, or TMD-related pain, (not to mention painful or cracked teeth), others may.

So, if you currently take one of these drugs AND have TMD, or have noticed an increase in bruxism, a different medication may improve your current headache or pain profile. Some people may be able to continue with the SNRI drug and add a medication called Buspirone, which can reduce the bruxism side effect with minimal potential for new side effects. This should be discussed with whomever prescribed the medication in the first place.

Increased bruxism is not the only possible side effect from SNRIs, others include: dry mouth, blurred vision, GI upset (diarrhea, nausea, constipation), drowsiness, insomnia (fluoxetine), sexual dysfunction, increase in suicidal thoughts, increased risk of bleeding especially if used with other meds that also increase bleeding such as aspirin.

The story can get even more troubling—people often seek additional prescription help for their TMJ pain, not realizing the medications they are already taking may be part of the problem. Prescription upon prescription can be a prescription for even more problems, because those people are now faced with the possible side effects of the additional medications.

Other drugs that can cause bruxism:
- Street stimulants (cocaine, ecstasy, methamphetamine). Please do not use these drugs for the sake of your family, well-being, teeth, and TMJs!

- Adderall—a stimulant used to treat ADD/ADHD

- Bupropion (Wellbutrin)—also used to treat Depression

- Alcohol

- Caffeine

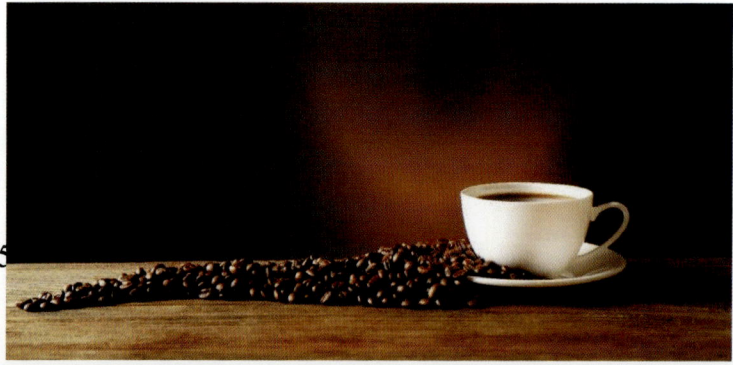

But wait, alcohol and caffeine aren't drugs!

Actually they are, *by definition*, and are likely the two most common drugs (also consumed legally) known to mankind.

It has also long been asserted by many in the dental profession that a bad "bite" can cause bruxism. While this controversy rages on in our profession, it seems more likely that bruxism may result in teeth damage but is not the root reason for the bruxism condition itself.

Those of us who manage TMD issues for the people that come into our offices can often manage symptoms, with great success. But I'm sure you'll agree with me that its always best to treat the ROOT CAUSE—which is one reason that our TMD patients who also have sleep apnea often get a "two-fer" from their dental sleep devices.

If you have active TMD symptoms and are currently using any of these medications, consider speaking with your prescribing provider about this issue (or give them a copy of this chapter/book). Finding the "right" medication for your mood disorder may also help improve your pain and long-term dental health!

7
Clenching & Grinding Your Teeth Might Cause…

So what happens when teeth aren't apart 99% of the time? If we now understand "normal" is teeth apart, then we can no longer say it is "normal" for people to grind or clench their teeth (perhaps you have been told this very thing at some point in your life). **Common**, yes! **Normal**, certainly not!

To understand this a little deeper, let's look at the definition of disease: *a disorder of structure or function, especially one that produces specific signs or symptoms.* Also we should note the definition of disorder: *a disruption in systematic function.*

Since clenching and grinding are not "normal", we can safely say they are a disruption of function (disorder), and they also produce very specific signs and symptoms (disease). Let's take a look at what clenching and grinding might cause.

Perhaps the most obvious effect of clenching and grinding is **premature tooth wear**. Research tells us the average person should "wear" their teeth no more than one millimeter in 100 years. Unfortunately, for those who grind their teeth one millimeter of wear can happen within a couple of years! Imagine if this was left untreated, what would be left of their teeth in ten, twenty, or even fifty years?

"Night guards" can help protect teeth from premature wear but may not be the answer (see chapter 17).

Another problem with grinding and clenching is **cracked or broken teeth and/or restorations** (crowns and fillings). Studies show when we are 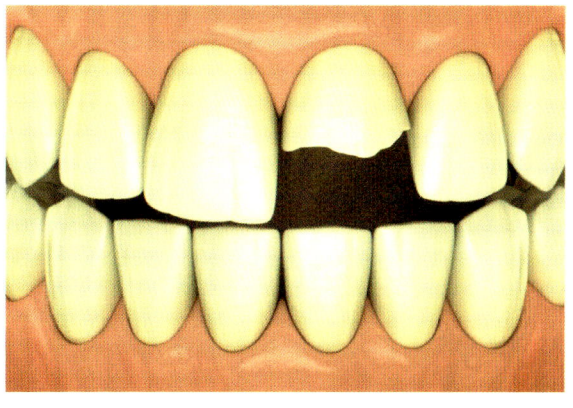 awake, we can put up to 250 pounds of pressure per square inch on our teeth. That's around 125 pounds, or about the weight of Angelina Jolie, on *one tooth*!

Unfortunately, it gets worse. When we are asleep, our pain receptors don't function the same and we can put up to 400 pounds of pressure per square inch on our teeth. That's 200 pounds of pressure on one tooth! Not only can this cause a lot of tooth pain, but it can also cause fractures and cracks in enamel, fillings, and crowns (caps).

Dentists reported an increase in cracked and broken teeth after 9/11, the Great Recession of 2008-10, and during the 2020 COVID pandemic. An increase of stress is likely the direct cause of this, as stress can be a cause of clenching.

Clenching and grinding can also cause **problems with our gums**. Gum recession is a common occurrence and happens from the extra force placed on the bone around our teeth. Bone dissolves when placed under pressure. So when we clench and/or grind our teeth over time that pressure dissolves the bone around our teeth…and our gums follow the height of our bone level. Voila— receding gum line.

Another issue that could be caused by clenching and grinding is called an **abfraction**. Excessive pressure can cause a loss of tooth enamel on the exposed part of the tooth along the gum line. The loss of tooth enamel creates a little wedge-like notch in the tooth which can sometimes be very sensitive to air and temperature.

If you think about the amount of muscle force needed to exude 250-400 pounds of pressure on the jaw, it's no wonder grinding and clenching also causes **jaw pain**. Pain in the jaw typically originates in the joint itself (directly in front of the ear) or in the various muscles in our face. These muscles range from our cheeks to our forehead, neck and back of the head. Most of the muscles in our head and neck are related to each other on some level (see chapters 1 & 4), and it's often surprising the areas of pain clenching and grinding causes.

Other minor signs of clenching and grinding show up in our mouth. Often people form a white or red callous line on the inside of their cheek (called **Linea Alba**). If this callous continues to get bigger it can make it hard to talk to chew without accidentally biting your cheek.

Another, and less often noticed sign is extra bumps of bone (called **Tori**) either under the tongue or along the gums on the top or bottom jaw. It is believed this extra bone is built up from abnormal forces placed on the bone from clenching and grinding.

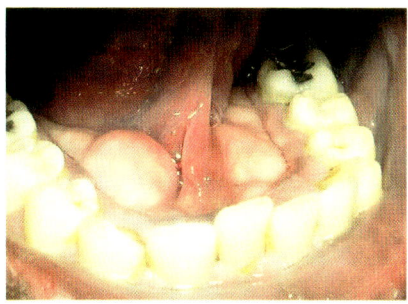

Perhaps you have some of these signs and symptoms of clenching and grinding? By now, hopefully you realize it isn't normal. In the next chapter, we'll discuss some other signs and symptoms that people might not realize could be related to clenching and grinding.

8

But Wait There's More!

Other Things Clenching & Grinding Might Cause

Did you know clenching and grinding might cause headaches?

Our jaws are very powerful! As just mentioned in the previous chapter, the muscles in our jaw can create a biting force of almost 250 pounds per square inch. Some experts estimate that this force can increase to 400 pounds of pressure of force per square inch when we clench or grind our teeth at night.

Clearly, this much force puts a great deal of strain and pressure on your temporomandibular joint (TMJ) and all its supporting muscles and ligaments. Your TMJ muscles span to your jaw, cheeks, and the side of your head. Thus, bruxism causes overuse to these muscles which can lead to throbbing headache pain, and in some instances, migraines.

But what are some of the other effects of teeth grinding and clenching? While for many people headaches may be the first, most noticeable effect of bruxism, others may notice earaches, congestion, ringing in the ear (tinnitus) and sinus pain because the TMJ muscles surround these structures.

Headaches occur more frequently in people with TMJ symptoms and can be divided into two main types: primary headaches and secondary headaches.

Primary Headaches

Migraine is a common disabling primary headache that is diagnosed on the basis of at least five attacks per month that last for 4 to 72 hours and are characterized by unilateral (one-sided) throbbing, moderate or severe pain accompanied by nausea, vomiting, sensitivity to light and/or sensitivity to sound.

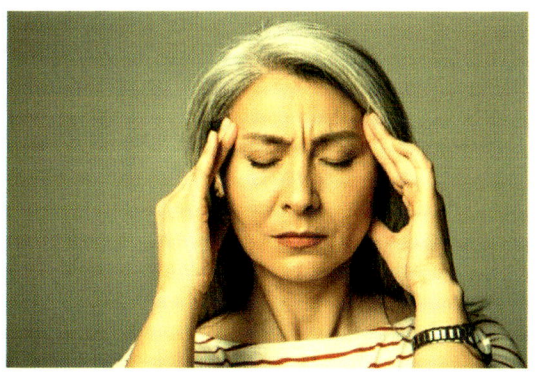

Migraine with aura is known as a classic or ophthalmic migraine and is diagnosed on the basis of at least two attacks per month, with symptoms including fatigue, difficulty in concentration, neck stiffness, sensitivity to light or sound, nausea, blurred vision, yawning and pallor.

Tension-type headaches are another primary headache that can be infrequent episodic or frequent episodic.

The infrequent episodic tension-type headache is diagnosed on the basis of less than 1 headache per month that lasts for 30 minutes to 7 days and is characterized by bilateral, non-pulsating, mild pain that is not aggravated by physical activity with or without head tenderness.

Secondary Headaches

Secondary headaches include **acute and chronic headaches** that occur after whiplash injury. Acute secondary headaches develop within 7 days after the injury and usually resolves within 3 months. Chronic secondary headaches also develop within 7 days after injury, although it persists for greater than 3 months.

Unstable jaw joint position and ear symptoms—is there a relationship?

TMJ disorders can cause various **ear symptoms**, including dizziness, ear ringing, stuffed eustachian tubes, and difficulty hearing. Although we don't always understand the mechanism, these ear symptoms are often part of a TMJ disorder. This is because they increase along with the other TMJ symptoms when the TMJ disorder becomes more severe, and they decrease along with the other TMJ symptoms when the TMJ disorder is relieved.

The balance mechanism, located in the inner ear, may also be affected. Severe injury to the balance mechanism results in dizziness and nausea. Mild injury to that same system produces feelings of disorientation, inability to concentrate, a tendency to bump into things, and "spaciness".

Tinnitus (ringing, roaring, or buzzing sounds in the ears) has been shown to respond to TMJ treatment in about half of the people studied.

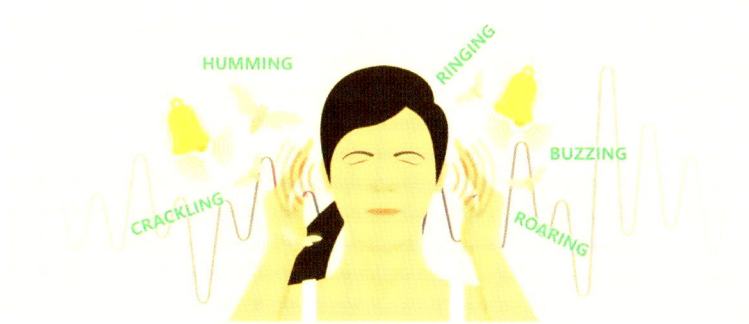

One cause of ear symptoms in TMJ disorders is probably inflammation of the retrodiscal tissues (remember those from chapter 3?). Anatomical studies of TMJ with dislocated discs have shown that most of the tissue bruising occurs at the extreme back end of the TMJ, located only 1.5 millimeters in front of the middle ear.

The increased fluid pressure that results from inflammation in that spot can transmit across the thin membrane bones separating the ear from the TMJ. Increased fluid pressure can also push the eustachian tube closed, which passes very close to the back of the TMJ. If it has been pushed closed for any length of time, it can become narrowed in that area. Subsequently it can be blocked by a cold, allergy, or anything else that causes inflammation of the inner lining of the tube and further narrows it.

A blocked eustachian tube can prevent it from equalizing pressure between the middle ear and the outside air and can create a stuffy feeling in the ear and difficulty clearing it after changes in altitude.

Another cause of ear symptoms in TMJ disorders may be the **loss of proper resting tension** in the two tiny ear muscles (the tensor tympani and the tensor veli palatini). Resting tension is the amount of "tightness" that a muscle engages even when it's resting and turned "off".

These 2 little muscles are controlled by the same nerve that controls the jaw closing muscles. If the TMJ tissue is damaged, that controlling nerve may trigger a bracing reflex to try to protect the TMJ, and as a byproduct also trigger that same reflex in the two ear muscles—creating an increase in the resting tension.

Increased resting tension in the tensor tympani muscle (the muscle that tightens the ear drum), can create subjective hearing loss which might be one reason a person with a TMJ disorder would complain they often miss things people say, even though hearing tests show normal results.

Increased resting tension in the tensor veli palatini muscles (which pull open the eustachian tube during swallowing), can interfere with the health and function of the eustachian tubes.

Some researchers believe that still another cause of ear symptoms being associated with TMJ disorders may be **Pinto's ligament**, which in scientific terms is a fibrous continuity between the sphenomandibular ligament and the anterior malleolar ligament of the middle ear (try saying that at parties…you'll impress everyone!). When we are born there is a tiny slit between these 2 structures that appears to close around the age of three, but some fibers may continue to pass through it and exert some pressure across it.

Whew! That's a lot of scientific talk. It all boils down to the fact that "TMJ disorder" is a complicated diagnosis with many symptoms that are affected by lots of intricate anatomy. Those symptoms are often very painful and disabling, and can create different headaches and ear symptoms (to name a few).

Gratefully, most symptoms respond well to conservative therapy if a correct diagnosis of the cause of the symptom is made. Managing the pain and restoring the range of motion in a TMJ disorder can improve the level of disability and often gives relief of primary headaches and ear symptoms.

9

What's That Popping & Clicking?

A Guide to the Common Noises in the Jaw Joint

Jaw joints can be annoying and pesky. They can prevent you from enjoying those big mouth burgers or get all the delicious goodness of a taco in one bite. Breaking up food that should be enjoyed together is a frustrating dining experience for anyone.

Your jaw joint and the noises that it makes. A guide to understanding those pops and clicks.

First things first, popping and clicking are anatomically the same thing. A pop or a click are not two distinct joint noises but are one in the same. It just depends on how the doctor, dentist, physical therapist, or you (the popper or clicker) choses to describe the noise. They are interchangeable.

Clicks (or pops) can be loud or soft. Clicks can also sound like a grinding or grating noise. The click can happen on both sides or more commonly just one, when you first begin to open or when almost fully open. The click can happen only sometimes or every single time you open your mouth.

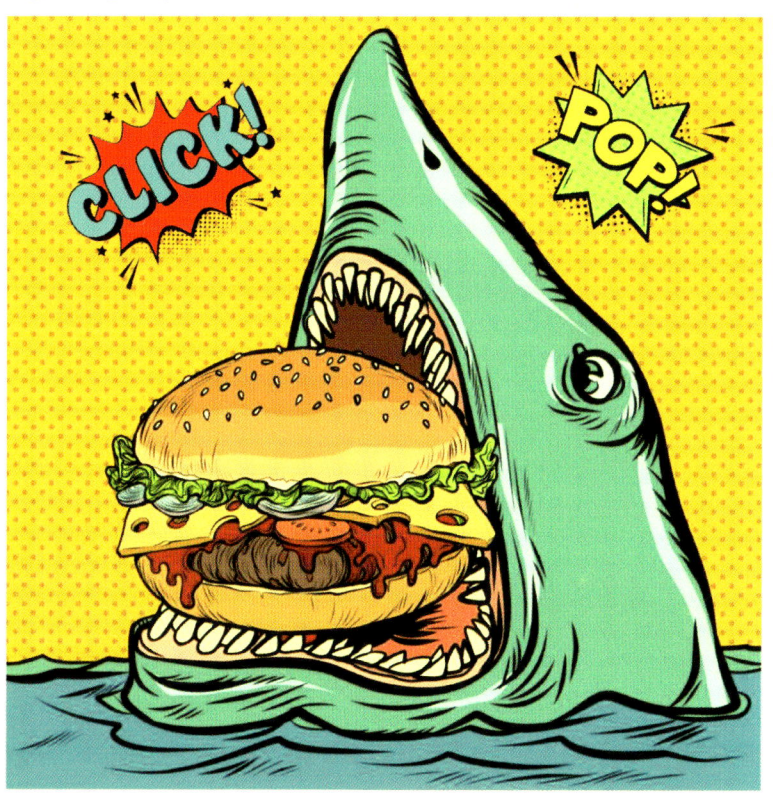

A **reducing disc displacement** is one of the possible causes of the joint noises that you experience. A reducing disc displacement is a long medical term that just means your jaw joint disc is out of place (dislocated) and then pops back into place. At rest, your disc is out of place and when you start to open your mouth it "reduces" or pops back into normal anatomical position.

If you've ever broken your arm you may have heard the doctor talk about needing to "reduce" the fracture. Reduction in this context means to bring back into normal anatomical position. Isn't it bizarre to realize that if you have a reducing disc displacement, your disc is out of place most of the time and it reduces **into place** only when you hear or feel that POP!?

If you think you or someone you know has a TMJ issue, try or recommend the following exercise, and answer these 4 questions:

1. Which side clicks or pops?
2. Is it early or late?
3. Is it loud or quiet?
4. Can you make the noise go away by changing your lower jaw position?

Question 1: Which side does your TMJ click/pop on? Sometimes you perceive a click/pop on one side, but if you place your hand on your face in a certain spot and open and close your mouth, you might notice that the pop is on the other side. The vibration through your skull causes the pop to feel like it's on one side when it's actually occurring on the opposite side.

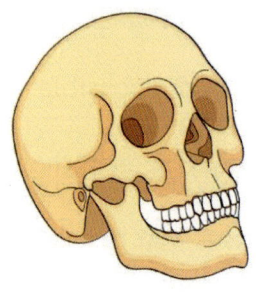

So place your hand near your jaw joint and open and close your mouth—where do you feel the pop? Now place your hand lower below the joint at the angle of your mandible (see picture). Is the pop still on the same side? Did it change?

Question 2: Is your click early (just as you are opening your mouth) or late (closer to when you are fully open)? Dentists will typically describe this as an **early or late click**. A late click means that your jaw is dislocated the majority of the time and there is only a small window at the end of opening where the disc pops back into place.

Question 3: Is your click loud or soft? Is it one distinct noise or a grinding type noise? A valuable point to understand about reducing disc displacements: the louder the click or pop **the better**. Weird I know, right? It might scare your dinner partner or your pets, but the louder the better.

In the anatomy chapter you learned about the shape of the disc and its purpose, and you got an overall view of the jaw joint.

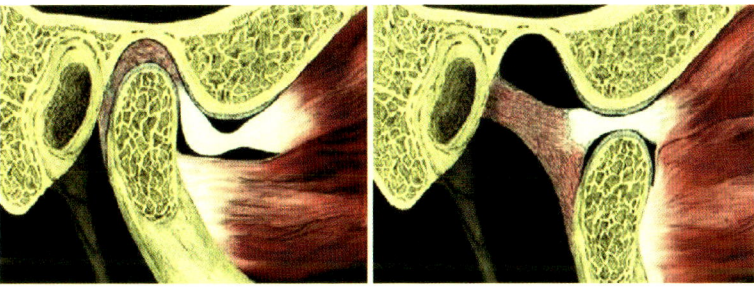

The disc clicking INTO place when you open is the noise you hear. Due to its hourglass shape, if the disc is healthy, the click will be loud. If the click is quiet, it typically means the disc has taken a beating over the years and is not the same shape it once was.

In the next photo, the far left shows a normal joint and, in the middle, a reducing disc displacement (clicking jaw). On the far right there are changes in the shape of the disc shown.

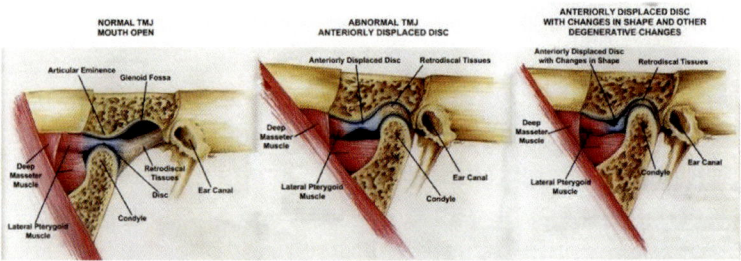

The joint noise starts off loud and then can become quieter overtime as the disc changes its shape. These changes are degenerative and are the cause of the noise changing from a loud pop to a grinding or grating noise known as crepitus.

Question 4: Can you make the noise go away by changing your lower jaw position?

Now for this last question, move your lower jaw forward and make your front teeth (top and bottom) touch each other. Open and close from that position (and return straight back to that position). Does the joint noise go away when you do this or is it still there? If it's still there, keep moving your jaw farther and farther out (like this bulldog/boxer mix pictured). Can you find a position where if you open and close the noise goes away?

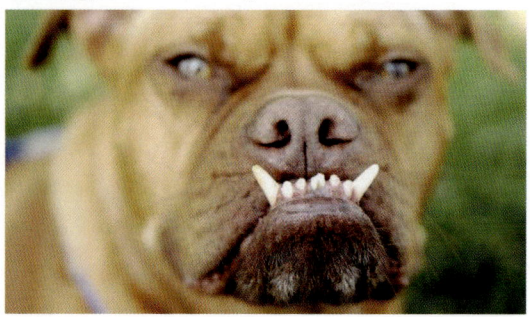

If yes, pat yourself on the back, you

have successfully found the position where your reducing disc displacement stays reduced (or stays in its normal, healthy position). If no, it might mean your jaw can't physically get to the position where your disc reduces, or it could mean you have an **eminence click** which is commonly mistaken for a reducing disc displacement even among health professionals.

Eminence Click

Normal mouth opening ranges from 38 to 52 mm, or 3 fingers stacked on top of each other between your teeth.

Opening more than 52 mm typically indicates hypermobility of the TMJ. Some will have hypermobility in their TMJ as well as in their other joints. The hypermobility allows the condyle to travel past the articular eminence causing a "thunk" type sound and the jaw may deflect to the opposite side.

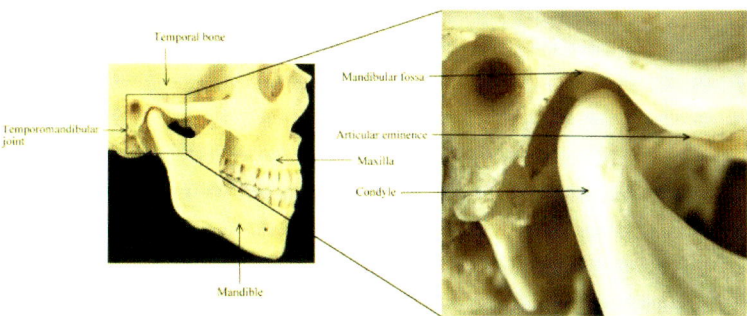

There is an easy test to see if your click is an eminence click or a true reducing disc displacement. Put your tongue on the roof of your mouth. Now only open as wide as you can while keeping your tongue on the roof of your mouth. If the "click" goes away, then it was most likely an eminence click and not a reducing disc displacement.

Exercise complete! Did you find out anything about your TMJ as you went through those questions?

Your noisy joint might be causing you some dysfunction or quality of life issues. It might not be an issue at all... besides scaring new friends when sharing a meal.

When treating these types of issues, the bottom line comes down to 3 things: improving your quality of life, alleviating dysfunction, and/or preventing future problems.

Determining a quality-of-life issue is subjective—only you can decide if you are being impacted by having noises and dysfunction in your jaw. If it doesn't bother you, then it's not affecting your quality of life.

If there are joint noises, we know there is some dysfunction in the TMJ. Your disc can turn from a loud noisy reducing disc displacement to a degenerative grating reducing disc displacement (more about who needs treatment in chapter 12).

In some individuals, after years of popping and clicking (and years of explaining their joint noises to dentists), their TMJ stops making any noise. Suddenly silence. What does that mean??? Did the problem finally go away? What a cliff hanger! We'll discuss what could be happening in the next chapter.

10

When the Clicking STOPS...
That's Probably Bad

Do You Have a Closed Lock?

In the last chapter, we talked about what it means when you hear clicking and popping in your jaw joint. It usually means your disc is out of place at rest and that it pops into place when you open wide. But what does it mean when the clicking stops?

Well, if you were undergoing TMJ therapy (which we will discuss in later chapters) for the displaced disc, then it's POSSIBLE that your disc went back into place.

However, when no treatment is done, then it would be *highly unlikely* that the disc could ever get back into place on its own. What's *MUCH MORE* likely is that the disc has moved so far forward out of place that it can no longer pop back into place when you open.

This dislocated disc is actually acting like a wedge, preventing the jaw from sliding down and opening all the way. Think of a doorstop that keeps the door from fully opening. That door can open part of the way but at soon as it hits the stopper, boom. Done. No more movement. It's as if the door is LOCKED at the halfway point.

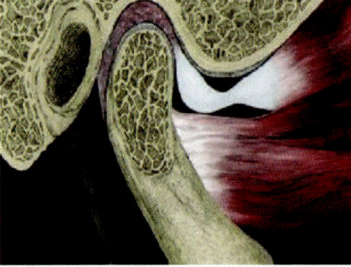 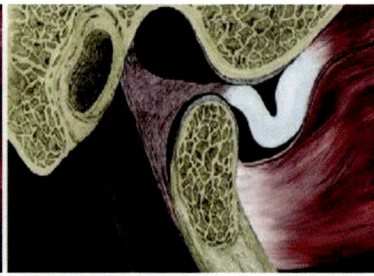

And guess what?!? When this happens to the jaw joint, we also say it's locked! The fancy name for it is a non-reducing disc displacement, but commonly we just call it a closed lock.

So what does it look and feel like when this happens?

Well, as mentioned above, the biggest sign is that the jaw won't fully open. It will rotate open about 26 millimeters, which is roughly the same as 2 fingers stacked on top of each other and put vertically between your teeth. No matter how far you try and stretch it open, it stops right at that same spot and just won't open any farther. You might think this would be painful but typically, it's not. It just feels really stuck. But it could be painful if you try to force it past the point where it's stuck.

The other distinguishing sign is how the jaw moves as it is opening. Normally, the jaw opens up and down in a straight line. When it's locked, the jaw moves off to the side where the disc is displaced and doesn't come back to the center. We call this "deflection."

So, you've got the 2 major signs of a closed lock: your jaw can't open past 2 fingers AND it deflects off to one side. But how do we KNOW it's locked FOR SURE? Do we even need to know for sure that it's locked and what difference does that knowledge make?

Well, if we catch it early enough, there is a good chance that we can UNLOCK the joint and get the disc back into place. We will talk about how a trained dentist can do that in chapter 17, but since it involves sticking a needle into your jaw joint, we want to know FOR SURE that it's locked before we do this.

The only way to "see" the disc and where it's located (or dis-located) is with an MRI. X-rays and CT scans will show hard tissue (the teeth and bones) but since the disc is made of softer and less dense tissue, we can't see it that way. An MRI will give an image of tissues of all densities and will show us not only the location of the disc but also information about the health of the disc and the joint as a whole. The MRI would also show us if there was something unexpected going on that's NOT a dislocated disc.

In the next chapter, we will discuss what it's like to have x-rays or an MRI on your road to helping your TMJ.

11

TMJ X-Rays & Imaging

What to Expect from a Patient's Perspective

As discussed in chapter 3, the TMJ is the hinge joint that connects your lower jaw, the mandible, to the temporal bone of your skull and allows it to move. Abnormalities in this joint can cause pain and discomfort in the muscle as well as joint dysfunction.

As discussed in previous chapters, **TMJ dysfunction** is a common condition and can be affected by many different things such as:
- Abnormal movements of the disc between the skull and condyle inside the joint
- Degenerative arthritis and inflammation
- Deposits of crystals in the joint and the soft tissue around them such as gout and calcium pyrophosphate deposition (CPPD)
- Very rarely: tumors (benign or malignant) and abnormal jaw shape

After your dentist does a thorough clinical exam, they may review their findings and order imaging for a TMJ problem, depending on your situation.

Reasons why you might need TMJ imaging:
- To confirm the disc shape and (mis)placement.
- To find the cause of persistent jaw pain.
- To evaluate an injury to your jaw or jaw joint.
- There are joint noises or tooth grinding with pain.
- A locked jaw is suspected.
- Screening for other conditions that can cause pain such as a sinus infection.

Depending on what your doctor thinks is going on, there are a few different types of imaging they can order for you.

Types of TMJ Imaging

Panorex

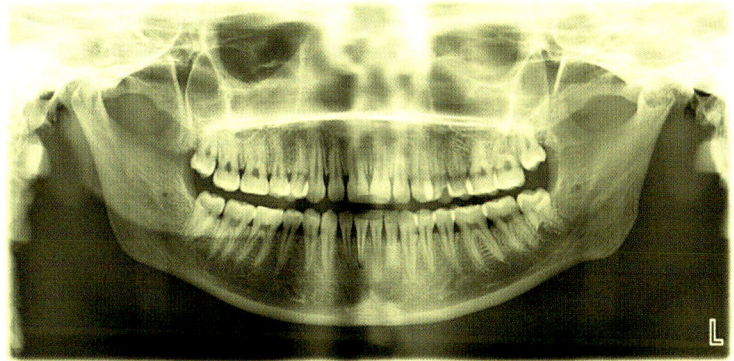

A Panorex is a great screening tool to see if there are condylar fractures (remember you have 2 condyles, one on each end of the jaw bone) or condylar head degenerative changes (arthritis in your jaw joint). This type of x-ray is a 2-dimensional view of the jaw.

Cone Beam CT
Produces a 3-D image of the skull, jaw and neck, including the airway. The teeth, mandible, TMJ, airway, sinuses, skull, and cervical spine (all the hard and boney parts of the head) are imaged in sections as well as in three dimensions.

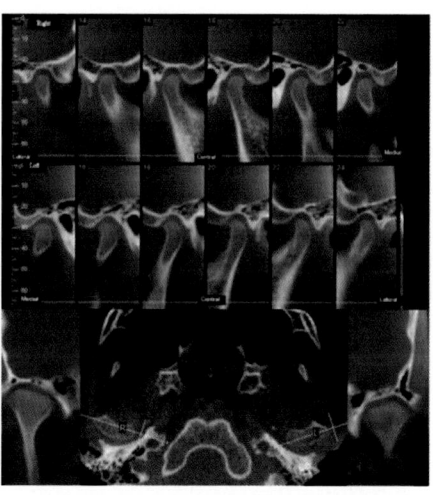

TMJ MRI
A magnetic resonance imaging scan (MRI scan) of the jaw uses magnets and radio waves to create detailed

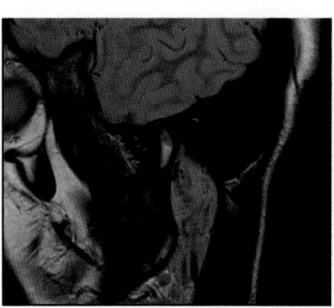

images of the soft structures in your jaw including determining the degree of swelling in the jaw joint. Looking at an open mouth and closed mouth view is necessary as well as other views. As discussed in the previous chapter, MRI's can be helpful to visualize soft tissue (like your TMJ disc).

Diagnostic Ultrasound
Diagnostic ultrasound for TMJ issues has only recently been used with only a handful of studies being done so far. These provide a sense of TMJ motion, the condition

of the top part of the lower jaw, swelling in the joint, and even disc position.

Your dentist will always be the one to determine which imaging or test would be most helpful in getting an accurate diagnosis. And remember, an accurate diagnosis is KEY to getting the correct treatment, which we'll talk about next.

12

Who Needs to Be Treated?

The PDQ Method

The PDQ method is something doctors and dentists often refer to when treating a TMJ problem. This acronym stands for pain, dysfunction, or quality of life issues (remember that from chapter 9?).

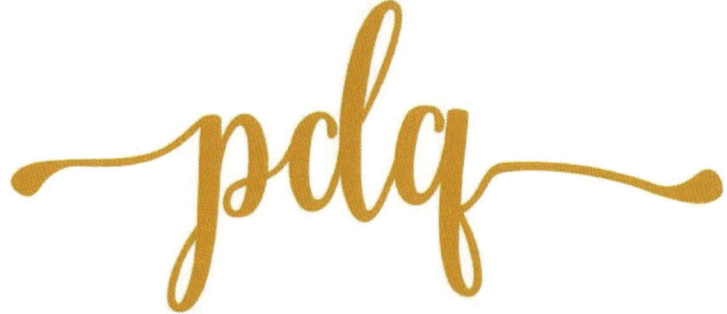

Different studies show that anywhere from 8 to 12% of the United States population is affected by TMJ disorders. Compare that to diabetes, which, according to the CDC, affects 10.5% of the United States population.

Eight to twelve percent of the United States population is about 35 million people. You are not alone!! But do all 35 million people with TMJ disorders need treatment? Not necessarily.

The classification of TMJ disorders is very broad and houses many types of symptoms, so the PDQ method was created to help decide who needs treatment. The caveat to this method is age. We will come back to this at the end of the chapter, but for someone who is young and has any sort of abnormal jaw joint, it is prudent to treat them using the original PDQ that I am sure you are familiar with—**p**retty **d**arn **q**uick!

Pain is often the driver of many treatments in the medical or dental worlds. Pain is an obvious reason to treat someone, but 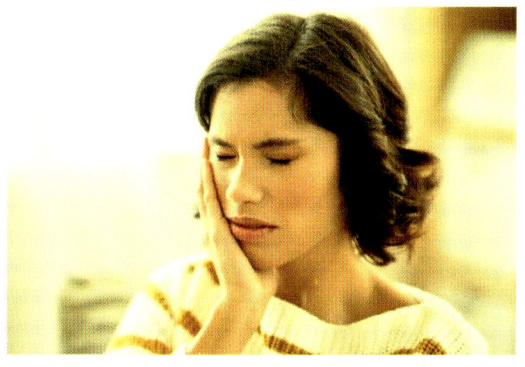 sometimes the source of pain is not always so obvious. Remember, with TMJ issues the site of pain (where you feel it) may not always be the source of pain, meaning where the actual issue is.

A recent patient of mine who spent three years seeing different ear, nose and throat doctors for what she described as a rubber band popping pain in her right ear. None of these physicians could find anything wrong with her ear and told her there was nothing they could do to help her.

Her dentist noticed that she also had a popping noise in her right TMJ so he sent her to my office. With the description of her pain, I concluded that it was possible that the site of pain was different than the source and I suggested that we attempt to treat her TMJ disc to try to alleviate what she perceived as ear pain.

Within the span of one week, in a TMJ orthotic, her pain of three years was gone. She had spent thousands of dollars seeking different medical opinions with no answers because her site of pain differed from the source of pain.

Why do you think that is? If you've read this book in chapter order, you can probably make a really good, educated guess!

When we spend the time understanding the anatomy, the wiring, and how our bodies function it becomes way easier to make a true diagnosis and get proper treatment.

Pain associated with the TMJ can come in different forms. Some people can clearly define the pain as pain in the joint itself. For others, the pain can be more difficult to describe.

As discussed before, our muscular and neurological anatomy is complicated and pain from the TMJ can radiate to different areas. You can have headaches, facial pain, perceived dental pain, and even neck pain all coming from the TMJ.

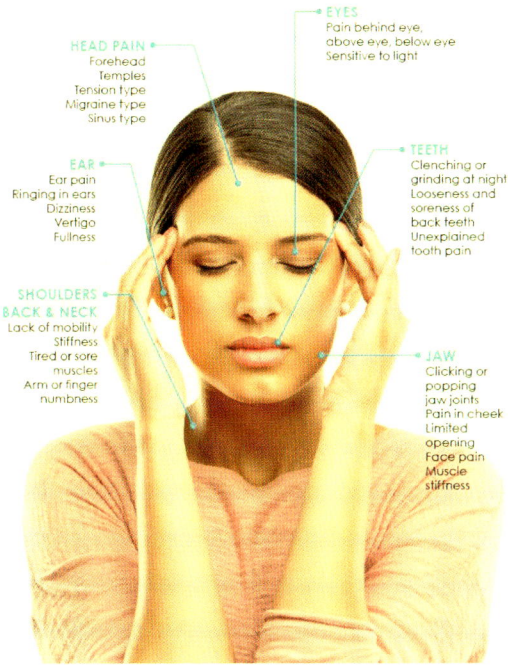

Dysfunction can be a relative term and is sometimes open to interpretation. For the purposes of this book, we are going to discuss proper function as being able to eat what we want, when we want.

Often people in our office suffer from a dysfunction called "the sandwich smash". They have to smash their sandwiches in order fit them into their mouth—they just can't open wide enough to fit the sandwich in otherwise.

Like discussed before, they commonly say, "My jaw used to pop, but then it stopped. Now I have to cut my food into smaller pieces or smash my sandwiches in order to fit them in my mouth." There may not be any pain in this scenario, but most people would love to function normally and be able to eat what we want.

Recently a patient came in who had chronic TMJ pain in both joints, but she told me she could handle her pain—she just wished she could look normal while eating at a restaurant.

While dysfunction can be a lack of opening, it can also be a jaw that doesn't move smoothly and uniformly. Remember, both TMJs have to work together simultaneously. For people who have a problem on one side, the jaw will often have to shift to that direction first before it can catch up to the other side and then it will shift back to the middle. For many people this dysfunction can be very uncomfortable, and even scary, when they must force their jaw either open or closed.

These types of dysfunctions need to be treated, because unlike a fine wine, they tend to get worse with time.

Now on to the "Q" in our PDQ...

One of the most rewarding parts of treating TMJ disorders is improving the **quality of life** of our patients. Most of us dentists and physicians have

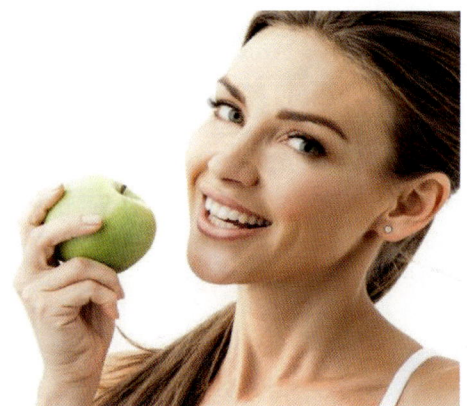

very limited training in the evaluation and management of TMJ disorders, and so people with these symptoms are often misunderstood and written off as overdramatic.

If you have gone for months or years with unmanaged pain or dysfunction, your everyday life will have to adapt in order to compensate. 'Quality of life' is the degree to which an individual is healthy, comfortable, and able to participate in or enjoy life events.

A young woman who had an injury to her right TM joint saw multiple doctors in her area over a six-month period and she had no resolution. This young lady then went to the internet and found a doctor who believed she could help her but unfortunately, was several thousand miles away. This doctor referred her to us, and she drove two hundred miles to be treated.

Within weeks, she was well on her way to returning to pre-injury status. Pain and dysfunction had now resolved but the young woman told me it had been so long since she had been social due to her condition, that she worried she wouldn't have friends that wanted to hang out with her anymore.

Her relatively common condition had motivated her to socially isolate herself for over a year while she had tried to manage her pain. She didn't want to be around others while complaining or not being able to eat normally. Her quality of life had completely changed and even now that she is back to normal, she continues to struggle to remember what normal was like. And unfortunately, this story is not unique.

The caveat to the PDQ method of deciding if treatment is necessary, is **AGE**. Like mentioned before, TMJ disorders typically don't get better with time. When a young person starts to have any TMJ issues, particularly youth that are still growing, it is prudent to treat the joints as soon as symptoms arise.

As the jaws continue to grow, they are designed to be on the discs. When growth is still occurring and the jaws are slipping on and off the discs, growth can be distorted and the negative results of this can be multiplied.

If you know a child or young adult who has **any** popping, clicking, or misalignment of the jaws please get them to a provider who can help as soon as possible.

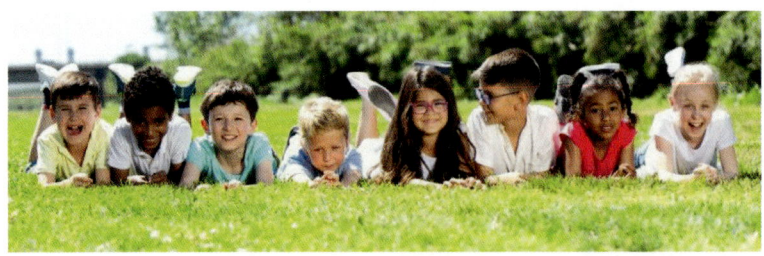

13

Treating Muscle Pain & Headaches

The Most Common "TMJ Problem"

Nearly everyone has a headache at some point in their lives. For some, the pain can be frequent, severe and even debilitating. Others may suffer from head and neck pain in addition to headaches. They may also experience problems associated with their jaw joints and the muscles that aid in chewing.

> *"Pain of muscle origin is one of the most frequent causes of discomfort about the head and neck." Weldon Bell, DDS – world-renowned author, lecturer and oral surgeon*

When you have a headache, you might not think that your jaw could be the cause, but one or both of your TMJ's could be the culprit. Headaches are one of the most common problems in people with TMJ symptoms. It can be hard to distinguish between general headaches and TMJ headaches.

As we all know from previous chapters, the TMJ is the hinge connecting the jaw to the skull. It enables us to do things like laugh, talk, chew and move the jaw side to side and up-and-down. Due to this hinging and sliding motion, this joint is a bit more complicated and can cause a variety of symptoms.

TMJ headache symptoms include jaw and facial pain, tight facial and jaw muscles, clicking and popping noises of the jaw, restricted movement of the jaw, and changes in the way the teeth fit together when biting.

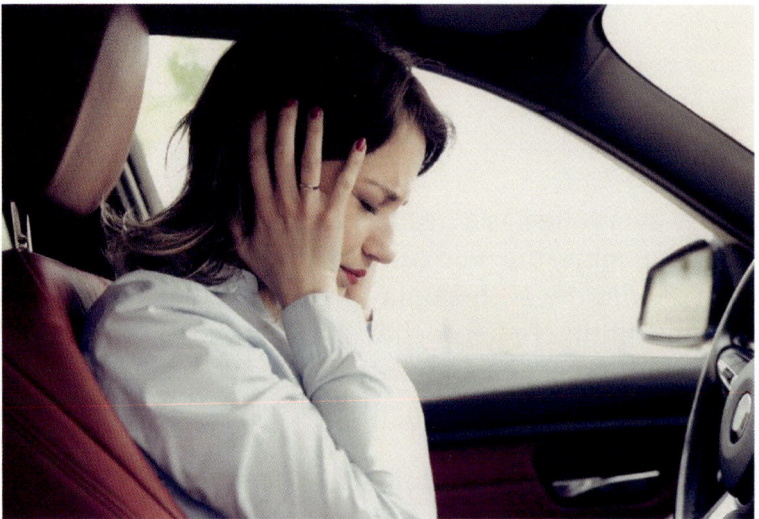

A few causes of TMJ headaches have already been mentioned but there are many more triggers that have been reported, like:
- Not enough rest
- Repetitive motion
- Repetitive muscle contractions
- Poor posture
- Dental problems
- Parafunctional habits like clenching and grinding of teeth
- Hunger
- Fatigue

- Dehydration
- Eye strain
- Low iron levels
- Alcohol consumption
- Smoking, and
- Cold, flu or sinus infections.

Since an accurate diagnosis is at the heart of every successful treatment, figuring out a solution for your headaches should always begin with a thorough conversation about your medical history, a comprehensive oral exam including muscle palpations of the head, neck and shoulders, as well as measurements of your range of jaw motion and most of the time some kind of imaging/x-rays.

Usually, the symptoms and pain are not a localized problem when dealing with the TMJ, but rather a condition that may affect the entire upper body. That's why it's so important to find a practitioner who understands the inter-relationships between the TMJ and head, neck and body pain. It's just obvious that finding the cause of your headache is essential to long term relief, right?

If the origin of the pain is muscular, there are therapy options to improve this condition. Initial treatment may include **a trial of nonsteroidal anti-inflammatory drugs** (NSAIDS). This trial will generally last for 4-7 days for the treatment of acute pain.

Additionally, a **temporary, water-filled orthotic** mentioned in chapter 5 might be used, especially if an "emergency" type therapy is needed. This little device is a great help in diagnosing and sometimes treating the origin of your temporomandibular joint (TMJ), muscle, and/or occlusal pain.

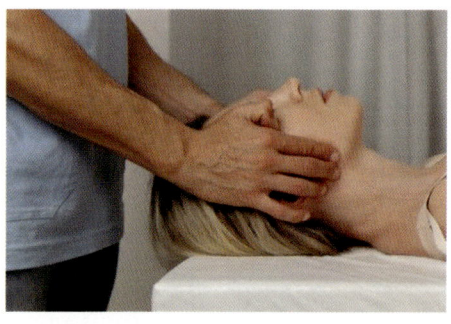

Physical therapy is another option. There are several specialized types of physical therapy that can help. Iontophoresis is a non-invasive treatment method which allows medication to be delivered externally across the skin to the painful area by way of a charged pad. Phonophoresis is another non-invasive treatment option involving the use of ultrasound to push medication across the skin. Low-level laser therapy (LLLT), also called cold laser therapy, uses low levels of light to stimulate healing in the affected area.

Have you ever heard of trigger points? If not, they are very tender knots located in a tight band of skeletal muscle. You can feel or palpate (press) them and produce localized pain and/or referred pain to another area of the head, neck, shoulders or body. This sore and improperly balanced muscle can even refer pain to other parts of the body. Thankfully they can be relieved with an injection to the knot of muscle that is the culprit of the pain. **Trigger point injections** relax the affected muscles and interrupt the nerve pathways that cause the pain.

Your doctor also might recommend the use of a **custom-made oral orthotic** as definitive therapy.

There are multiple other non-drug pain management techniques available, including **acupuncture**, **chiropractic care** (done by a chiropractor who understands the complexities of TMJ pain), **biofeedback**, and **cognitive behavioral therapy** (CBT). That last one, CBT, is a behavior modification therapy and might include areas of stress reduction, sleep hygiene and elimination of parafunctional habits such as pencil or ice chewing, and teeth clenching and grinding.

Finally, beyond the initial trials of NSAIDS, other medications that may be used to treat the pain include muscle relaxants, benzodiazepines, antidepressants, anticonvulsants, steroids, and Botox injections (more on those in the next chapter).

It is always better to treat the cause of the problem and not just the symptoms. Selecting a dentist trained in TMJ disorders can establish a safe and reliable treatment plan that can reduce headaches and enable you to chew, open your jaw and even sleep better. Since many people with TMJ symptoms also have symptoms of sleep apnea, don't be surprised if your dentist talks to you about your sleep quality! If your headaches and jaw pain are caused by sleep issues, then both of these conditions should be treated for the best results.

How wonderful would that be—no more pain AND better, more restful sleep!?

14

You Probably Don't Have a Botox Deficiency

If you have been reading this book in order, you've come across chapters describing the TMJ anatomy, causes and diagnosis of TMJ disorders, and possible management of TMJ pain.

In this chapter, let's review one of the management options you might have heard of—alleviating TMJ pain using Botox injections.

While there is no doubt that Botox injections can be effective in reducing pain, many physicians, dentists and researchers are concerned about this short term, Band-Aid-like solution being used for everyone and for all kinds of complex TMJ cases. Is Botox really a one-size fits all solution? Does diagnosis really have nothing to do with long term solutions to TMJ symptoms?

A lovely lady came to our office complaining of poor sleep and morning headaches. Her request was to have

Botox for her headaches as her friend was getting the injections and it "worked great for her".

A thorough, comprehensive examination and history revealed a few interesting things.

She did indeed have many symptoms (some of which she didn't even relate to her poor sleep and headache issues):

- She woke frequently at night and could not return to sleep,
- She had daytime fatigue and sleepiness,
- She couldn't focus well while at work,
- Her teeth had begun to wear down,
- She reported a crown was placed on one tooth after it had cracked,
- She reported she woke up with morning headaches, and they often persisted through the day,
- As we were speaking and doing her examination, she had trouble relaxing her jaw and her teeth were constantly touching together.

We began to put the puzzle pieces together. We discussed each symptom and sign. We discussed "common" doesn't mean "normal", we talked about how muscles, joints and teeth out of harmony cause issues and that she indeed

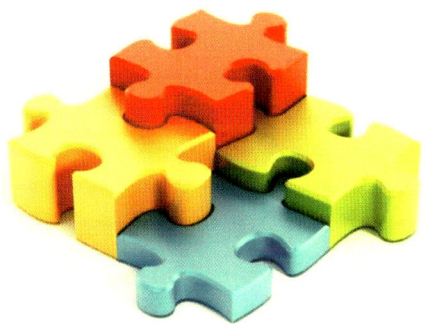

had a sleep issue.

Then we discussed the option of Botox, as she did come in for that treatment after all. Botox can be used for a number of things both cosmetically and medically.

For cosmetics, you are probably aware that Botox can indeed reduce facial wrinkles. It does this by blocking the nerve conduction to the muscles of the face, paralyzing the muscles, so they can't contract thus no wrinkles on the skin.

Many men and women have this procedure done for cosmetic purposes and which is wonderful if that's important to them. It was first approved for cosmetics in 1989 but it really gained popularity after it was developed into a commercial product by Dr.'s Jean and Alastair Carruthers in Vancouver, British Columbia, Canada. They called it "Botox Cosmetic."

For medical purposes Botox has some wonderful uses, especially in the field of spastic muscle disorders such as cerebral palsy, post-stroke spasticity, post-spinal cord injury spasticity, and several other conditions involving muscle spasticity which are debilitating and severely effect quality of life.

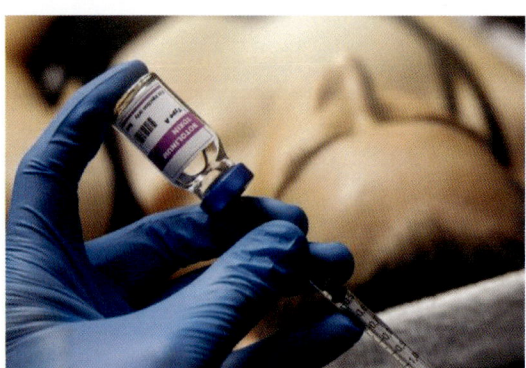

But what exactly is Botox, and should it be of used for headaches and "TMJ"?

The long medical answer is that Botox is an inert version of "Botulinum Toxin," a neurotoxic protein produced by the Bacterium Clostridium Botulinum. There are 7 types of this toxin of which 2 types (A and B) are used to treat various muscle spasms in humans.

And the short answer is Botox is an injectable serum that can reduce muscle contractions that cause tooth grinding, tooth clenching and headaches (due to strained muscles).

But the question remains, just because you can, does that mean you should?

Obviously, the benefits of less muscle pain, limited tooth wear, alleviation of headaches and the bonus of fewer wrinkles can be attractive. But the reality of this band aid procedure is that Botox could actually be covering up the cause of those issues, creating more issues (especially if you have sleep apnea), and is not a long-term solution or cure for most TMJ problems.

There are also several downsides or possible side effects to Botox, such as:
- Weakening your chewing muscle strength
- Creating unwanted paralysis such as droopy eyelids
- Can be very costly as it often needs repeat applications every 3 months (between month 2-3 the effects can begin to fade)
- If you are clenching or grinding your teeth at night to protect your airway due to sleep apnea, you could make your sleep apnea worse by paralyzing those muscles.

In the end this sweet lady, headache and all, decided to look more at the cause of her pain rather than just masking the symptoms.

- She did a sleep study which confirmed the presence of obstructive sleep apnea.

- In the management of her sleep apnea, with a custom oral appliance, we were able to improve her sleep quality. We reduced the number of times she woke through the night. When she did wake, she could usually fall back asleep easily.

- Her morning headaches significantly improved, her daytime fatigue and sleepiness reduced, her ability to manage stress improved and her ability to focus and recall topics at work improved.

- She became more aware of her daytime stress levels and how she was managing, or mismanaging, the stress.

- She began learning and implementing mindfulness and relaxation breathing techniques which helped her stay calmer and manage situations better.

- And after we had discovered and treated the cause of her symptoms, she decided to do some Botox for purely cosmetic reasons—which in her case was the right reason.

For TMJ, Botox can be a temporary stop gap or a trial treatment possibility or a treatment of last resort but managing the true cause of the TMJ pain and dysfunction should always be the first goal.

The reality is that a TMJ condition is not a Botox deficiency. If you want to use Botox cosmetically or have any of the muscle spasticity conditions, it can definitely help and those are great uses for it. Just be wise and informed when you decide to get rid of a few wrinkles.

15

Sprains Aren't Just for Ankles

Ligament & Tendon Issues

The Mayo Clinic defines a sprain as a stretching or tearing of ligaments, which are the strong bands of tissue that connect two bones in a joint. They also define tendinitis as the irritation or inflammation of the tissue cords which attach muscle to bone, or where the muscle inserts into the bone.

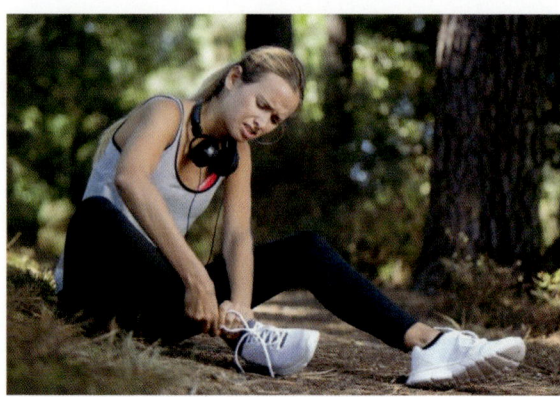

Most of us have experienced sprains, strains, and tendinitis types of things during our lives. If you have, it was probably in your wrist or ankle—the most common place for those types of injuries.

But did you know you can sprain your jaw? Did you know you could develop tendinitis in your TMJ?

As we've learned, the TMJ can be very complicated, but it is still A JOINT. Thus, the usual injuries we experience in other parts of our bodies can also happen in the jaw. We do not usually think of it that way since we don't run or walk with our jaw joint, or train it to endure a particular sport...

Or do we?? Have you "trained" your TMJ muscles, ligaments, and tendons to function a certain way without even knowing it?

The most common of these types of injuries to the TMJ is called "temporal tendinitis." As we learned in chapter 4, the temporalis is a big fan shaped muscle on the side of the head that inserts into mandible (or jaw bone) right under and beneath your cheek bone. This injury, then, is an inflammation of the area where this important muscle inserts into the bone.

How could you possibly develop tendinitis in this spot? The temporalis muscle is used to elevate your mandible...or in other words to close your mouth. Maybe your friends weren't joking then when they said you talk too much....

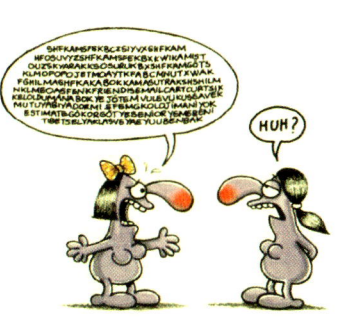

A frienD is...

...someone who listens to you

...or maybe, joking aside, there is true trauma to the area. A car accident, a ball to the side of the face, or even the habit of clenching the teeth cause trauma to this ligament by overusing the muscle.

Do you still have all your back teeth, or have you had molars removed? As the muscle works to lift the mandible, the teeth are what stops this movement. This means having missing teeth could start an imbalance in the function of this muscle and the health of its attachment to the bone.

So how do you know you have temporal tendinitis? What are the symptoms? Pain in the tendon is the biggest symptom, of course, but pain in the head easily radiates to more places and so sometimes people will feel a pressure in their ear, discomfort near their eye, or pain around their upper back teeth.

If you're thinking to yourself, "I have those symptoms!" then what can you do about it?

By now, you should agree, that first things first, we always want to figure out WHY something is happening before we treat a problem. It's better to find causes before treating symptoms, as it produces better, longer-lasting results.

If the TMJ trauma is due to a habit like clenching, a custom daytime orthotic can be worn to give biofeedback to the muscles and hopefully create a new, healthier habit.

If the problem is from muscle overuse due to missing or worn-down teeth, replacing and restoring a proper bite can maintain a healthier muscle.

If there was an accident creating the injury, anti-inflammatories, injections, and physical therapy may be the way to go.

Ernest Syndrome is a "sprain" of the jaw that can occur when the stylomandibular ligament is injured. This ligament goes from the temporal bone of the skull to the lower corner of the mandible and its job is to prevent the lower jawbone from drifting too far forward.

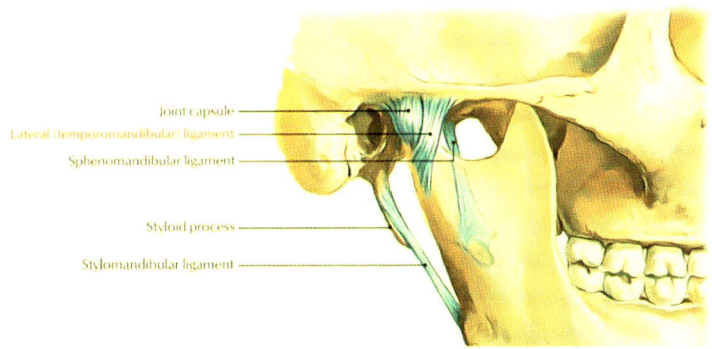

This injury can be a result of whiplash or car accidents and trauma, but is sometimes difficult to diagnose as the pain is transferred to multiple areas. Similar to temporal tendinitis, the pain can often be felt as a fullness or pressure in the ear, tenderness near the eye, the joint itself or even under the cheekbone. But Ernest Syndrome develops into additional discomfort into the throat and the mandibular teeth (your bottom teeth) instead of maxillary or upper teeth like temporal tendinitis.

Because these injuries can feel so similar, your dentist will usually confirm the diagnosis with an injection of anesthetic and a small amount of steroid directly at the place where the stylomandibular ligament inserts into the mandible. This often resolves all symptoms of Earnest Syndrome but if it doesn't, working with a pain management physician that can perform radiofrequency therapy is very valuable and can usually help you avoid unnecessary larger surgeries. Radiofrequency therapy works by "turning off" the smaller sensory nerves that are hypersensitive to the injury.

It is clear that the source of jaw pain is not always the joint itself. As with all other TMJ challenges, these sprains and strains usually require a deep dive into sleep or breathing issues and/or muscle patterns to see if they may be contributing factors.

Do you snore all night long? Is your brain trying to keep your airway open? Are you grinding and clenching your teeth all night? Remember trauma can be created by overuse of muscle and ligaments. Muscles of the head and neck working too hard during the night to avoid obstructions in breathing can result in trauma.
A thorough medical history and diagnostic sleep study can help to ensure the reason behind the pain or injury is addressed properly so that we are not just treating the symptoms, but truly solving the problem.

One of the simplest and most effective ways to stabilize the healthy muscles of the head and neck is working on your posture. Our modern lives are full of smart phones, iPads, and computer-work which almost always leads to a head position that is pushed forward and dropped down. This puts an unnecessary and harmful amount of improper force on our cervical spine which causes our head and neck muscles (including those of the TMJ) to become imbalanced, compromising stability and thus causing trauma.

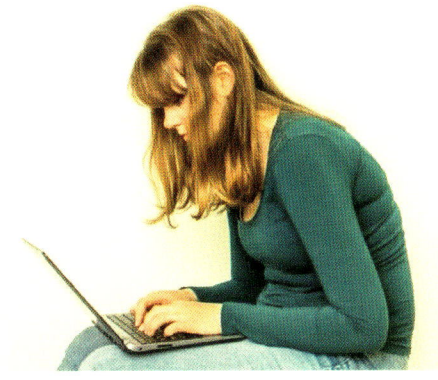

This illustration of a cervical retraction exercise is one which we often jokingly call "the double chin stance" and works to correct the imbalance a forward head posture creates. It is a simple thing you can do at home, takes a short amount of time, and is hugely beneficial to strengthen proper posture.

Mckenzie neck exercises:

Head retraction: With proper upright posture, slowly retract your head (with chin tucked) as far as possible, hold for 4 seconds or so and relax. Rest and repeat for 10 repetitions (per session). Perform 6 sessions spread out evenly throughout the day.

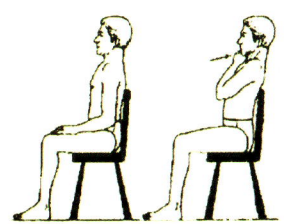

If the cervical spine is aligned properly, the muscles of the shoulder, neck and TMJ can then function in harmony. Strain on structures like the temporal tendon and the stylomandibular ligament can be eased while improper overuse can be minimized and even breathing, whether during the day or while asleep, will be more efficient.

"The first step towards change is awareness" said psychologist Nathaniel Branden. Try being aware of your head and neck posture during the day and when you catch yourself, correct it and see if some symptoms start to resolve over time.

16

Treating Popping & Clicking

Why a Dental Term Called "Centric Relation" is Important to you

A good friend of mine, when he was in dental school, spent most of his little free time playing basketball. He remembers finally finishing his mid-term exams during his freshman year. He had buried himself in the library cramming as much gross anatomy, biochemistry, and pharmacology into his head as possible in a week. When exams were finally over, he was itching to get back on the court.

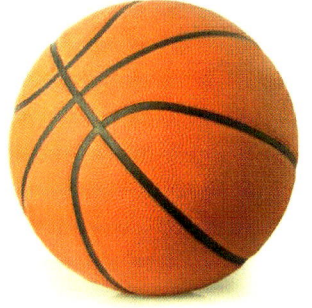

He rounded up his dental school classmates, and they were off to the gym. He was not an exceptionally talented basketball player, but he made up for it in blocks and rebounds. He told me that he vividly remembers the other team's player missing an easy shot, but he got his own rebound, and was about to make a layup. With all my friend's pent-up energy from exam week, he jumped hard and high to block the other player's next attempt. As if in slow-motion, as soon as my friend jumped the other player ducked and he went flying over him. Before he knew it, he had landed on his shoulder and fell in a tumbled heap. He knew something was wrong—he couldn't even help himself up. All the muscles around his shoulder seized up immediately in pain.

He made it to the emergency room suspecting a dislocated shoulder. After what seemed like hours and hours of waiting in pain, the doctor finally made it to his bed. He couldn't wait to have the doctor relocate his shoulder. As the doctor inspected his x-rays, he confirmed that my friend's shoulder was dislocated.

And guess what?! The first thing the doctor did was to attempt to relocate my friend's shoulder. That makes sense, right? But what if the doctor had just recommended some ice and heat, or perhaps a massage or ultrasound, with a good measure of rest. Would that have helped? Would it be smart medicine to just treat the muscles around the shoulder joint without putting it back in place first? Of course not.

Isn't it weird that the TMJ is the only joint in the body where most doctors and dentists tend to ignore a dislocation—where the disc is out of place? Instead, we simply treat the muscles around the joint. Although a dislocated shoulder is not completely analogous to the temporomandibular joint, it's interesting that we treat the TMJ differently than any other joint in the body.

Similarly, the temporomandibular joint may undergo a traumatic event such as whiplash from a motor vehicle accident or simply from your overexcited child knocking his head into your jaw. This trauma may loosen the tight ligamentous fibers surrounding your joint capsule allowing your disc to slip forward. As you recall from previous chapters, the little hour-glass shaped disc is supposed to be between the condyle (the ball part of the joint) and the glenoid fossa of the skull (the socket).

We've talked about popping and clicking in chapters 9 and 10, but let's take a closer look to really help us understand those bizarre noises (most dentists don't even fully understand why your joints are making noise).

Although we may not experience a traumatic accident to our jaw, many of us induce daily "microtrauma" to our jaw. This microtrauma is usually from clenching and grinding one's teeth together.

We've already talked about the forces we can put on our teeth. Remember the 250 lbs. per square inch of force we talked about? When we clench or grind our teeth, we should be concerned with the forces placed on them. Dentists may point out "wear facets" on the top surfaces of our teeth as they are flattened out over time.

However, there is an equal amount of force applied to the other end of the jaw. Imagine all that force distributed among all 32 teeth also being focused on two spots, the right and left temporomandibular joints. Similar to stepping on a bar of soap, this pressure can cause the disc to slip forward.

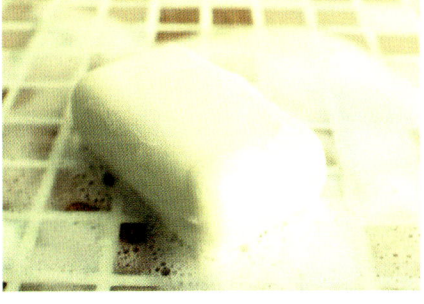

107

Consider automobile accidents—the everyday microtrauma from all that force of clenching and grinding your teeth from the *emotional* stress AFTER the accident can cause more cumulative harm on the joint than the motor vehicle accident itself.

When the disc slips forward, it can no longer act as a shock absorber, resulting in degenerative changes or breakdown of the joint. Over time an x-ray or CT scan may reveal that both the ball and socket part of the joint have flattened out.

Now that the disc has slipped forward of the joint, otherwise known as an anterior displacement, the disc must relocate back onto the joint to allow the mouth to fully open. Another way to think about the function of the disc is as ball bearing. The disc, or ball bearing, needs to be on the joint for it to fully open. As you open your mouth, the disc will relocate or reduce back onto the joint. You will usually experience this phenomenon as a click or a pop. Then when you close your mouth, you will experience another, usually quieter click or pop. This clicking noise is the disc slipping forward again out of the normal anatomical position.

WHEN DO WE TREAT THE CLICKING DISC?

Although we gave a rather graphic illustration of a dislocated shoulder joint, it has been our experience that not everyone with a clicking temporomandibular joint needs to be treated.

Going back to PDQ, we would not treat someone who does not have any pain, dysfunction, or quality of life issues related to their TMJ. For some people, a clicking joint can be stable without causing any PDQ issues for years. For other people, a clicking or popping joint might be a progressive step towards issues in the future.

But if you are in pain, have trouble eating due to the joint catching or locking, or are simply embarrassed at the dinner table from a loud popping noise with every bite, we might consider managing your symptoms by attempting to bring your joint into more physiologic position known as centric relation position.

WHAT IS CENTRIC RELATION, AND HOW DO WE GO BACK TO IT?

Centric relation is the normal anatomic position of the disc properly placed between the ball and socket portion of the temporomandibular joint. This position allows the disc to act both as a shock absorber and a ball bearing.

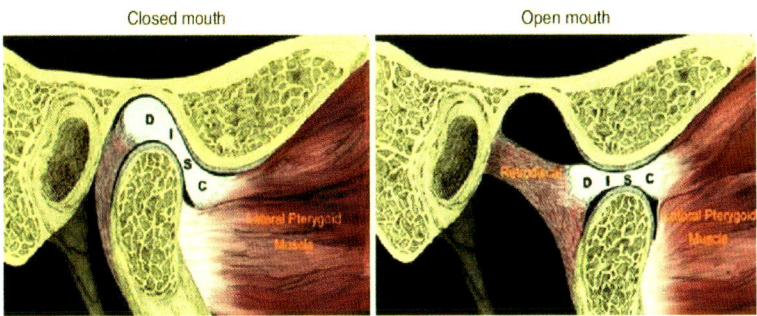

If the disc is displaced and clicking, your TMJ provider will make you an orthopedic repositioning device that you wear on your teeth. This orthotic is similar to an orthotic in a shoe. It's only functional is to guide your foot into the correct anatomical position as you step into it. Similarly, the orthopedic repositioning device of the jaw joint gently guides the mandible forward as you close your mouth.

Guiding the jaw forward will allow your disc(s) to stay in "centric relation," the normal anatomical position between the joint and socket. These orthopedic repositioning devices can be made for both nighttime and daytime use.

MY DENTIST ALSO RECOMMENDS THAT I CHANGE MY BITE WITH BRACES OR CROWNING ALL MY TEETH.

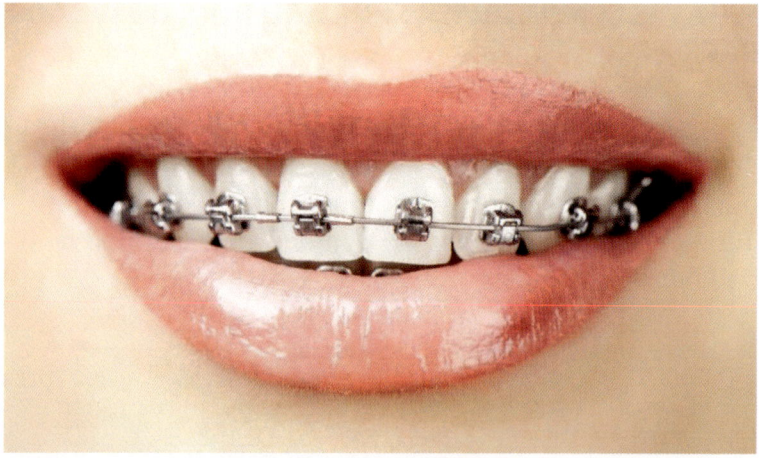

When a dentist recommends changing your bite with orthodontics or crowning every tooth, it's usually called phase 2 therapy (the use of the orthotic repositioning devices I just talked about is referred to as phase 1 therapy).

The goal of phase 1 therapy is to provide the patient relief from pain. Phase 1 therapy is usually achieved with the use of removable orthotic devices. However, if you wear the orthotic repositioning devices long enough, typically greater than 6 months, this continuous use may create a new bite position as the muscles around the temporomandibular joint permanently adapt. The thought process behind recommending phase 2 therapy is to make permanent the new bite position that got you out of pain in the first place.

If you slide your jaw forward, you will notice that your upper and lower back teeth may no longer touch as you bite down. Phase 2 therapy will involve either orthodontics or placing crowns on all your natural teeth to make your upper and lower teeth meet up again.

Although this type of therapy may be necessary for some, in our practice we have found that we can wean almost all our patients off the daytime wear and avoid permanently changing our patients' bites.

The secret of our successful weaning is "the 1% occlusion rule". As mentioned in chapter 5, the best position for your jaw joint is to have your lips together and your teeth resting apart—only creating contact between your teeth when you swallow or chew (1% of the day).

We can achieve the 1% occlusion rule with the help of wearing the orthotic day and night.

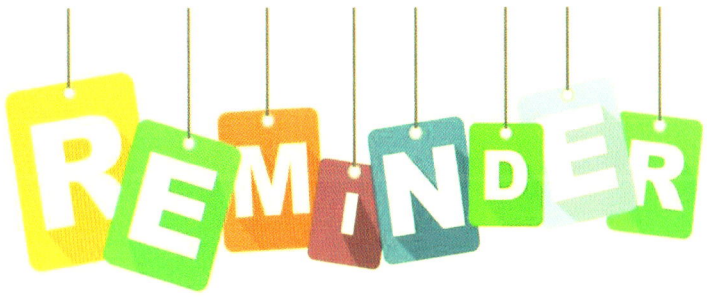

During the day, the orthotic will protect your joint when you bite down, but it will also serve as a behavioral reminder to keep you from clenching or grinding.

While you are sleeping, your doctor can't wake you up to tell you to stop clenching and grinding your teeth together. And even if they could, you would just go back to sleep and start clenching and grinding again. But with nighttime wear, the orthotic positions your jaw in centric relation, we can keep the disc in place when you clench or simply swallow while you're sleeping.

The centric relation orthotic allows your disc to heal and stay in place to serve as the shock absorber and ball bearing you need. And hopefully it will also keep you from having costly and invasive dental procedures.

17
Your Clicking Just Stopped & Now You Can't Open?
Do This NOW (and DO NOT Do This)!

Last night you went to bed, and everything was "normal". Your jaw was clicking or popping, as it has done for a long time, and you could still open your mouth fully. Now you wake up and you can't open your mouth anymore. It's actually stuck! What the heck do you do now?!?

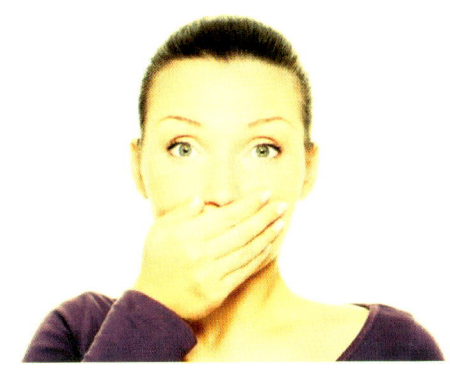

Looking back to chapter 10, this is the classic presentation of a closed lock, or non-reducing disc displacement. The disc has moved so far forward out of place that it can't pop back into place when you open. You likely can only open your mouth 2 finger widths and your jaw deflects to one side when opening. This may or may not be painful, but it is definitely alarming.

Time is of the essence! The sooner you get help for a closed lock, the more likely you are to successfully get unlocked.

The first thing to do is call a dentist that specializes in TMJ disorders. They will see you for a consult and then likely order an MRI to confirm that the joint is, in fact, locked (remember that X-rays and CT scans can't show the soft tissue of the disc so an MRI is the only way we can see where it is).

Once the disc position is confirmed, a TMJ dentist will have you come in for an "unlocking procedure." That could sound a little scary, but it's relatively quick and simpler than you might think.

Here's how it works...

Since the disc is wedged out of place, we need to create a space to allow it to pop back into place. A small amount of short acting anesthetic (the normal numbing medicine used for regular dental procedures) gets injected into the jaw joint space between the condyle and your skull. This fluid increases hydraulic pressure in the joint and makes a little space for the disc to get back into the right spot.

Once the anesthetic fluid is in the space, we start to slowly move the jaw around. This gentle manipulation helps increase that joint space even more and hopefully the disc will slide back into place. Depending on the joint, sometimes 2 injections are needed to get enough fluid into the space, especially since the anesthetic carpules only hold a little fluid (less than 2 mL) each.

So how do we know when the disc is back in place?

There are a few signs...
- First, the jaw joint will start popping again when you open your mouth.

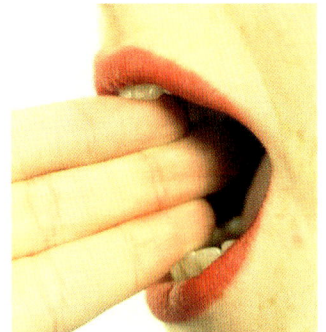

- You will also be able to open wider, likely 3 finger widths instead of the 1 to 2 from before the unlocking procedure.
- Your jaw will also open in a straight line instead of deflecting to one side.
- The last sign is that the teeth won't come together normally on the side where the injection was given. This is due to the fluid increasing the joint space. This extra fluid will get absorbed and metabolized by the body within a day or so.

Hooray! Now that your joint is unlocked, how do we KEEP it unlocked? As soon as you bite your teeth together, the disc will likely get wedged out of place again, resulting in the joint locking back up (just like it did before). This means we MUST keep the teeth from biting together.

We accomplish this by using a custom orthotic that fits on your lower teeth. It gets set in a specific position so that when you bite down you bite on the custom orthotic and not your natural teeth, keeping the disc in the correct spot all the time.

You will have to wear this orthotic 24 hours a day for at least the first 4 days. That means eating, drinking, talking, and sleeping with it in place. It will feel a little weird, but you adapt to it quickly. If the orthotic isn't worn, the joint will lock up again and you'll be starting over from scratch with another unlocking procedure.

After the first 4-7 days of wearing the custom orthotic 24/7, you will then take the orthotic out only during meals.

We've talked about what to do if you find your jaw locked, but there are a few things you should FOR SURE AVOID...

Do NOT:

- Wait to seek help. The sooner an unlocking procedure is done, the higher the success rate.
- Go to a chiropractor or physical therapist. These therapies have their place but not for a locked joint. Stretching or joint manipulation can actually wedge the disc further out of place, thus making unlocking LESS likely to be successful. In the unlikely event the chiropractor or physical therapist gets the disc into place, it will just slip out and lock up again as soon as your teeth come together.
- Do your own stretching exercises, risking wedging the disc even further out of place.

- Get a regular night guard over the counter or from a general dentist who isn't trained in TMJ therapies. These can both make the problem worse—you need to make sure you have an orthotic that is holding your disc in the right place, not the wrong place.

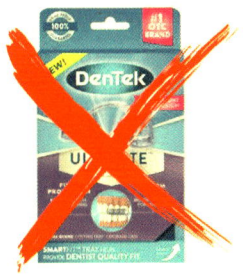

- Start orthotic therapy, orthodontics (braces), or let a dentist grind on your teeth without an accurate diagnosis and treatment plan in place.

- Ignore it, hoping it will go away or get better on its own.

- Freak out...there is help available!!

When a closed lock is diagnosed early, the odds of successfully unlocking the joint are high, as long as you get in to see the right TMJ dentist quickly.

18

Why a Nightguard Might NOT Work for You

A Strange Connection Between Sleep & TMJ Problems

"You are grinding your teeth and ruining them!" exclaim dentists around the country. "You need a nightguard to protect your teeth!"

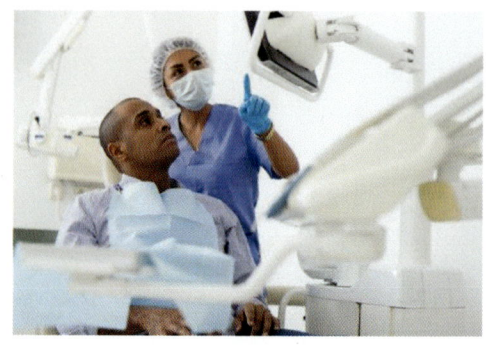

Was this you at your last cleaning or examination appointment? You might have been told by your dentist that you have evidence of bruxism (grinding or clenching your teeth, as discussed in earlier chapters). Maybe your dentist even recommends a "nightguard" to help minimize the harmful effects of your nighttime jaw jiving.

So why do people grind or clench their teeth especially while they sleep? We have lightly covered some possible reasons in previous chapters, but I'd like to address 4 of them in depth:
1. Stress
2. A joint problem (i.e., displaced disc)
3. Sleep apnea
4. Posture—does it play a role in this?

Here we go!

Stress

When people experience stress in their lives, they can respond in several different ways.

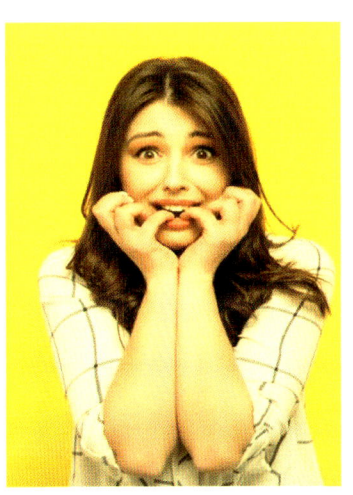

One, almost default response for many, is to put their teeth together and clench or grind their teeth. As discussed previously, this coping mechanism can lead to an overabundance of muscle activity.

The muscles of the jaw, neck and shoulders prefer to be in a rested (not contracted) state. Remember that muscles can only be in one of two states: 1) rested and relaxed length or 2) contracted, shortened length. They prefer the rested state because it requires less energy from the body.

A joint problem

The excessive muscle activity could be the result of a **displaced disc** in your temporomandibular joint.

The displaced disc can be likened to having a pebble in your shoe. As you walk, the discomfort of putting your full weight on that pebble triggers an avoidance behavior; so, you start putting more weight on the foot without the pebble. If you walk long enough, your poor positional gait causes your back and side to hurt.

When a disc is displaced, it may be difficult for the muscles of your jaw and neck to exist in the much-desired resting state. If you are avoiding chewing on the side of the displaced disc, this could lead to utilizing muscles that you would not ordinarily use just to avoid the pain.

Sleep Apnea

And yet a third explanation for why people grind or clench at night is a condition called **sleep apnea** (a sleep breathing disorder in which a person stops breathing when they're sleep). We've talked about stress and TMJ problems in other chapters, so let's explore sleep apnea...

When a person stops breathing at night (sleep apnea) it's usually because their airway collapses and the body can't inhale. The result is a state of oxygen deprivation. The brain is not a happy camper when there is an oxygen shortage, so the brain will go into survival mode to get oxygen and it tells the heart "Hey heart! Wake up!"

There is an adrenaline rush message from the brain to the heart that kicks your body into a fight or flight mode. This is an excited state that the body doesn't like to exist in. Some people wake up with their hearts racing as a result of this adrenaline.

Sometimes the brain figures out that by moving the jaw forward, the airway is opened and breathing resumes. Oxygen deprivation, especially to the brain, can automatically cause the TMJ and the muscles around it to contract. This constant muscle activity causes tension in the TMJ as it is attempting to keep the airway open. Hence the clenching and grinding.

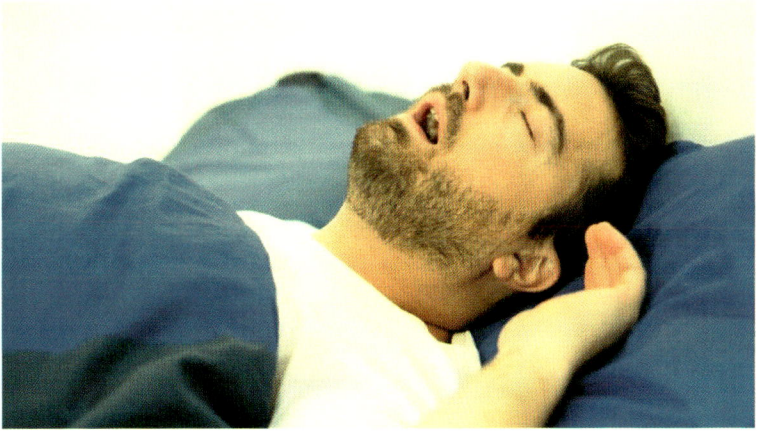

Sleep apnea is diagnosed by a sleep study. If you've had one of those, you may have gone to the sleep lab to spend the night. You were "wired up" to measure a whole host of body functions like heart rate, snoring, body position, the number of times you stopped breathing, etc.

It's interesting that when sleep doctors interpret sleep studies, the data will oftentimes show a large increase in jaw muscle activity. This activity is a measure of your clenching or grinding. So, you are sleeping and breathing normal, then suddenly you stop breathing and attempt to restart breathing several times; you initiate grinding (muscle activity), which results in finally catching your breath. This pattern repeats itself over and over throughout the night.

The conclusion is that the clenching or grinding of the teeth helps to open the airway. Well, if your airway is continually collapsing all night long and you are grinding all night long to open it back up, your jaw muscles and joint may be very tired, tight, and exhausted in the morning.

An oral appliance for sleep apnea addresses the airway blockage by keeping the jaw from falling backward, and research has shown that this treatment can substantially reduce bruxism (grinding and/or clenching). So, the oral appliance helps you AND your jaw get a restful night's sleep.

On the other hand, a night guard doesn't stop you from grinding or clenching. In fact, it only minimizes the wear on your teeth. A nightguard doesn't address the degree and amount of you are grinding, it just lets you destroy the plastic instead of your teeth.

Most dentists also don't realize that some types of nightguards could make sleep apnea WORSE!
A 2004 research study showed that "flat plane" upper nightguards increased sleep apnea events by more than 50% in half the participants. (Flat plane nightguards typically fit on your upper teeth and are smooth against your lower teeth so they slide easily—these slippery devices take away the one thing your brain is using to

keep you alive and breathing at night...the ability to hold and tighten your jaw to keep your airway open!)

You can see why it is crucial for everyone to be tested for this life-threatening disease before using a nightguard.

Posture

Way back in chapter 1 (and several after that) we've mentioned posture affecting your TMJ as well as your other head and neck muscles. Often a postural examination is performed when being evaluated for a potential TMJ problem.

Our anatomy is so complicated and connected that there are times when a **postural problem** can lead to a jaw imbalance and those jaw imbalances might also result in grinding or clenching.

These are just 4 of the possible causes of bruxism. There are probably many more!

It's key that we understand WHY you might be grinding or clenching in order to offer the correct treatment.

If you have bruxism because of stress, then a common nightguard will protect your teeth. But if you are clenching or grinding your teeth because of a TMJ problem, a postural issue or sleep apnea it's likely a common nightguard won't help much and may even make your condition worse!

19

No, You Probably Don't Need Braces or All of Your Teeth Crowned

You Need an Accurate Diagnosis and Conservative Treatment

Good news! You probably don't need surgery or super expensive dental work or orthodontics! As we've said over and over, what you do need is an accurate diagnosis and appropriate treatment.

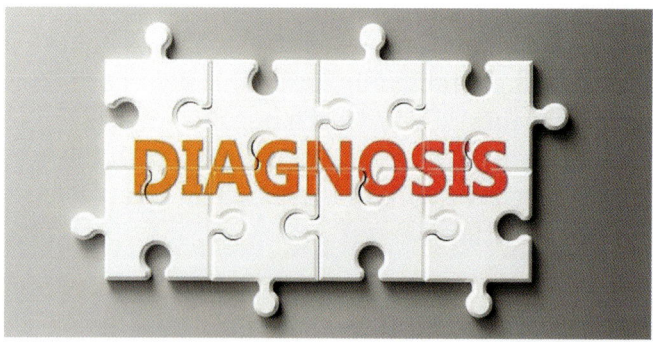

Knowing is half the battle! Effective treatment cannot be given unless there is an accurate diagnosis. First thing to do is set up an appointment with a dentist who has specialized training in TMD.

If you are considering a dentist that advertises TMJ therapies, make sure they:

- Do a comprehensive TMJ exam involving a thorough history of the problem, current symptoms and measurements of the jaw as well as any previous treatment for the problem.
- The dentist or one of their team members should ask you many questions, including questions about how you sleep.
- During the exam, the dentist should observe how your mouth opens and closes, and feel the joints and muscles of mastication (chewing muscles).
- In more complex cases, arriving at a diagnosis may require an MRI, diagnostic injections, cold therapy, and/or a temporary splint.
- They will probably talk about OPQRST in relation to your pain & symptoms:
    - **O**nset of pain/symptoms—when did it start? How long have you had them?
    - **P**rovoke & Palliate—is there anything that makes the symptom better or worse?
    - **Q**uality—describe the symptoms' characteristics (dull, throbbing, stabbing, burning, intermittent etc.)
    - **R**egion—point with one finger to where it hurts most

- **S**everity or Scale—on a scale of 0-10, where 0 is no pain, and 10 is being burned alive, where is your pain?
- **T**iming—when do you usually feel the symptom, how long does it last?

Before your first appointment many people feel it's helpful to make a list of things that improve the discomfort or symptom and things that worsen it. Keeping track of the above OPQRST will help you and your doctor come to a clearer diagnosis.

Do NOT take pain medication before the exam as it can interfere with getting to the root of what's really going on.

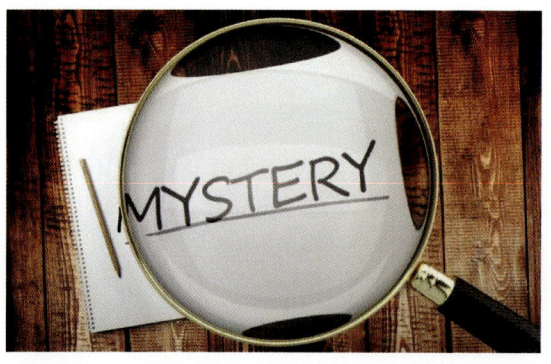

Arriving at an accurate diagnosis can be like solving a mystery. As we've discussed many times, the TM joint is very complex, and the symptoms can be complex and varied as well. The doctor will be collecting clues when they are talking with you and performing their examination. Once all the evidence is in place, they will hopefully be able to identify the cause and not just the symptoms.

Once you have an accurate diagnosis, therapy can be correctly directed (not just masking it with medication or a nightguard, but helping you get relief from your real issue). Most of the time you don't need surgery either! Conservative therapies should always be the first step. If that does not solve your issues, consider surgery as a last resort.

What is conservative therapy? There are many types of conservative therapy and what is appropriate obviously depends on the diagnosis. These are a few of the most common:

1. Ice, moist heat, over the counter pain medication and a super soft diet. You have probably already tried these things, but really committing to them for 5 days can make a huge difference.
2. Orthotic therapy—worn during the day and night. These orthotics place the jaw in a position to decrease pain and prevent and sometimes heal damage to the joint.
3. Physical therapy with a specially trained therapist can greatly reduce muscular pain that does not respond to other treatment. If you and your dentist decide this is necessary, ask for a referral to a specialist that has the appropriate training.
4. Trigger point injections can provide fast and lasting relief.
5. Joint injections using PRF, or anesthetic followed by joint stabilizing orthotics.

The risks associated with conservative care are minimal. The biggest risk is doing nothing because the outcome is further deterioration and pain.

20

Being a Dental Instrument For Mankind

Unlike so many people, I liked going to the dentist. Crazy, I know, but I fondly recall my visits going to the dentist as a child. He was a German dentist, who was born in Nairobi, Kenya but had gone back to Germany for his schooling. There was always something about him that I admired, and it was clear that he loved his work. As I got older, he began talking to me about becoming a dentist. He must have sensed my interest.

I was always good with my hands too, and I loved the idea of helping others. So, I decided that I too was going to be a dentist.

After graduating I was your typical drill, fill, bill dentist. I was happy. But there was something missing.

Once our son was born, my wife started suffering from severe migraines and tension headaches that on some days, left her incapacitated. She started taking multiple medications and having lots of doctor visits.

Medications would give her some temporary relief, so she was able to take care of our children. Sometimes I would have to come home early from work if she was having a really bad day.

An orthodontist friend of mine suggested that perhaps her "bite" was contributing to her headaches. So she started orthodontic treatment.

Amazingly, her headaches started to subside during the treatment, and she began feeling better. While I was discussing my wife's transformation with another colleague, he suggested that it could be that her jaw joint was the problem and that the orthodontic therapy may have been repositioning not just the teeth, but the joint as well.

Apparently, her TMJ was contributing to her headaches and the bite shifting was making the TMJ better. We had not been taught about TMJ and the headache connection in dental school. Few dentists even today, understand the relationship. Fewer physicians do as well, which is why so many people take medications for headaches.

After the orthodontic treatment was finished, the migraines and headaches came back again. I remember times when she would seclude herself in a dark room with absolute silence. The children became aware that Mom was not feeling good and in her room, and knew to play amongst themselves, silently. It was a hard time for us as a family as we had to adjust to how my wife was feeling on a day-to-day basis. Mom's headaches impacted the entire family!

I felt helpless not being able to help her fix the problem permanently. I started going to all her doctor visits as well, to help find a solution for her. The medications were only taking the edge off the pain.

I would have discussions with the various doctors about TMJ and the possible headache connection, and they were all sure that TMJ had nothing to do with her headaches and that they were truly just migraines and only medication would control them. This wasn't good enough to me though—there was a consistent nagging in my head about the TMJ connection and it continued to bother me. I decided I had to find out about TMJ and its connections.

This started my journey into TMJ. I decided that I was not going to learn from only one doctor or system but from multiple doctors and systems. I did not want to have "one hammer and one nail" for treatment. As it turned out, I tried a lot of different treatments on my wife before she was finally freed from her headaches.

My wife has now been headache free and off all medications for 30 plus years.

I have a lot of mentors to thank along this journey; Doctors: Brendan Stack, Peter Dawson, Farrand Robson, Dan Gole, Mike Mazzocco, Bob Walker, Terry O'Shaughnerly, Roger Melkonias, Jeckman, Larry Funt, James Carlson, Holstrom, Bill Hang, Jamison Spencer, and Michael Goldberg.

Along this journey I have completed a lot of education in chiropractic and osteopathy. The jaw doesn't function solely by itself...it is attached to the rest of the body. These courses helped me learn how the body/muscles work. Ascending problems come from the feet, descending problems come from the teeth, and everything in between needs to work in harmony to have optimal health.

In 1995 I read about a Canadian Dentist, Dr. Holstrom, who had fallen asleep driving and hit a tree. The damage was so bad, he was lucky to have survived. He developed a snoring and sleep apnea appliance so he could treat himself. I took his courses and from the other mentors previously mentioned.

When chronic pain patients get rid of their pain, their lives, and the lives of those around them change as well. Many of them get rid of depression, for they have a much better outlook about the life. Similarly, when patients start getting better, more restful, and refreshing sleep, they and their families have similar experiences. They are more productive and energetic. Other, associated health issues improve, and their overall health improves.

It's amazing how freeing a person from pain or poor sleep can free so much more!

For the last 15 years, I have dedicated my career exclusively to treating TMJ, snoring, and sleep apnea patients. The feeling of satisfaction we get at my office when patients come back pain free and have slept soundly through the night is completely overwhelming. We get appreciation and hugs every day for changing their lives in such monumental ways.

Our mission is to change lives. My motivation is to help my patients become pain free, well rested, and enjoy an excellent quality of life. My reward is when people come back and are overwhelmed with joy on how their lives have been changed for the better.

One person at a time.

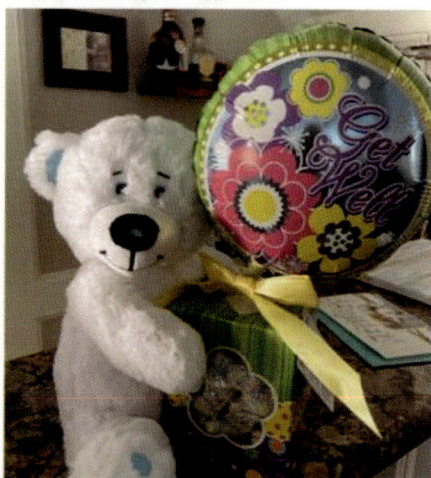

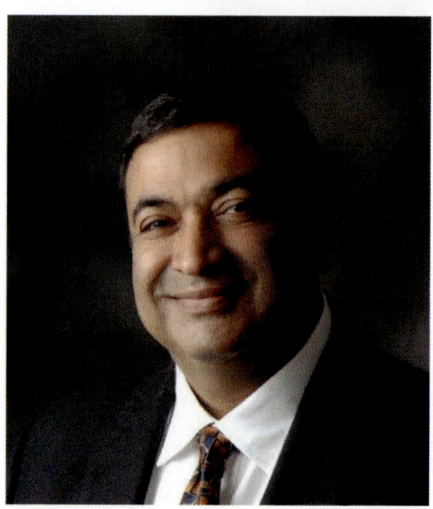

21
Real Life Patient Stories

"Leaving my appointment with my new appliance I thought, "how is this going to help my pain?! It's a piece of acrylic", but I was wrong. My everyday headaches, ear ringing, and aching pain are a thing of the past. Don't wait and adapt to your jaw pain, it won't get better on its own. Take a chance and get your life back. I was very sore for a week after my teeth/jaw adjusted to the appliance. Don't give up on it and in 2 weeks' time, you'll realize you underestimated Dr. Patel's appliance and I owe him great thanks. He's awesome!"

--Janine G.

"I've had this trauma for over 10 years. Some years good and some bad, but when the trigeminal nerve pain kicked in, I knew something was odd. I did convince a doctor to do an MRI and he found a compression and I had MVD surgery. After surgery, I went back to work and the pain came back after 3 months. They wanted to burn the nerve next, but I thought that wasn't curing the problem. I found Dr. Patel and his crew on Google and was admittedly skeptical at first. The cost worried me, that it would be another expensive treasure hunt. I gave them a shot and have absolutely zero regrets! First week of the appliance, the pains were subsiding but still present. Second visit, second adjustment and I've been zero pain for the last 3 weeks. My biggest request to the

Dr and his wonderful crew was if they could help me get my life back...and they did! This crew knows what they are doing. God Bless them."

--Anthony R.

"After one and a half years of facial pain that went through my ear and down my jaw, I was having intense headaches on top of that. When pain grabbed me, I had to take off my glasses and grab my face. I couldn't even talk during these episodes, and pain was going down under my tongue. Finally, I found relief after visiting Dr. Patel. He made me a custom orthotic that took pain away and helped reduce my seizure medicine that I probably didn't need to begin with! On my way to a healthier, pain free life... thank you Dr. Patel!"

--Sandra B.

"I strongly recommend Dr. Patel, as I can't believe how his treatment has helped my mother's facial pain that she has suffered with for over a year. No medications helped her until she started with treatments under the care of Dr. Patel. I'm so grateful that she made the decision to follow his treatment plan as she is now almost 100% pain free. Very grateful for Dr. Patel and his staff. Everyone is so kind and nice!"

--Shelly S.

"It's crazy what one week can do, going from dealing with TMJ for 10+ years to getting no pain in one week. I had to call off work due to pain from my jaw and migraines 3 to 4 times a week....imagine going from that, to having just a small headache once in the entire week. I'm so thankful I was able to get help without surgery. I thought I was stuck being in pain for the rest of my life."

--Itzel F.

"The week I came in I was in so much pain that I was crying myself to sleep. I hadn't had solid food in over a year and I could barely fit a teaspoon in my mouth without dislocating my jaw. My first week with my device I had my pain reduce from a 9-10/10 to a 3-4/10 consistently. I'm able to fully open my mouth and eat solid food again. I no longer have to hold my jaw in place when I eat, brush my teeth, yawn or laugh! My quality of life has improved so much, it's hard to even put into words!"

--Constance M.

"When I was about 8 years old, I started have what my parents thought were ear problems, that occurred every time I would open my mouth to eat. But my doctors always told me it was nothing serious and I trusted that conclusion… until I was 15 and trying to get braces, and I had to be sent from doctor to doctor until I came here and Dr. Patel explained what was wrong. After starting his treatment, I noticed my mouth started to open much more than it could before. My headaches were not bad anymore and my jaw clicking is not as frequent. This treatment has really been helpful for me, considering how long I have had this problem. The results are very quick too and I would recommend it to anyone with the same problems."

--Brigette C.

"I came into the clinic complaining of migraines that seemed related to facial pain concentrated near my jaw. I was immediately relieved when they provided me with such a sound solution. I was able to do a fitting for my jaw device and very soon after I started wearing it, my pain has reduced drastically! I'm so grateful to have found a solution for my pain so quickly. The team of people here are so friendly and kind. I immediately felt taken care of. Thanks so very much Suburban TMJ & Sleep Center!"

--Auni D.

"I can't believe the difference one week made for me. Dr. Patel took the time to listen to me, and didn't make me feel rushed during my appointments. After the first week I was shocked at how much wider I could open my mouth without pain. I had no idea how much my jaw way affecting other areas in my head and neck. My only regret is that I waited so long to make an appointment with Dr. Patel. If you are on the fence, go for it! It truly is life changing within a matter of days! I am very grateful for Dr. Patel!"

--Amy F.

"I was sent to Dr. Patel by my dentist for TMJ. Dr. Patel also found that I had sleep apnea. My jaw, teeth, neck and head now feel great with the TMJ fix. I wake up in the morning without headaches from the sleep apnea. Thank you for all the help."

--Brian R.

"In one week my TMJ pain went down to practically zero. Device was made quickly; instantly reduced my pain. Doctor and assistants were great. Doctor followed up the next day himself just to make sure I had no pain and that the device was comfortable. Highly recommend them to anyone with Jaw/Dental pain."

--Mike S.

"After over a decade with chronic pain and headaches being brushed aside by my primary doctors, finally was recommendd to see Dr. Patel and cannot pass along the recommendation enough! Within one week, my pain I

have lived with for half my life was gone and I am now as close to normal as I can be. Dr. Patel and his whole team have been wonderful and sincere throughout the whole journey, and I owe them much more than I can ever give. Thank you to Dr. Patel over and over again."
--Laura B.

"I was having chronic headaches and a lot of jaw pain. With the splint from Dr. Patel, my headaches have subsided, the pain in my jaw is gone. I am able to have a more normal and pain free life, thanks to the help from Dr. Patel and his staff. I am grateful that the splint has worked so well and that I was finally able to find the causes of my pain after visiting countless doctors and specialists, none of which were able to pinpoint TMJ as the <u>true</u> cause of my issues."
--Sydney C.

"I came to Dr. Patel two weeks ago and received my oral appliance. My jaw pain has almost completely reduced and every day it gets better! Adjusting to the appliance is the hardest part, especially with your speech. However, the benefits greatly make up for that slight inconvenience. I'm so glad Dr. Patel was able to find the source of my jaw pain and get me on the road to recovery!"
--Mary M.

"I came to Dr. Patel unable to eat or open my mouth. (I couldn't eat tortilla chips or anything like that). My pain was unbearable, it was keeping me up at night and affecting my diet. After a few short weeks, my pain is almost nonexistent. Last night I ate pizza without a struggle. I can open my mouth again. It's been such a drastic and complete change. Dr. Patel helped me so much and I couldn't be happier with my results so far."
--Yuvia S.

"I'm so grateful to Dr. Patel for his knowledge and experience that helped me progress so much in just one week! The appliance he made me is very comfortable and is just what I needed to relax my jaw and correctly align my bite again. I don't want to ever be without it! I am so excited to continue to progress with his care! My pain, popping and clicking has been greatly reduced! I was nervous to pursue treatment because I didn't want anything to make things worse for me. Didn't have to worry about anything with Dr. Patel's treatment, he was what we had prayed for!!!"

--Tamara G.

"Before I came to Suburban TMJ and Sleep Center, I had constant jaw pain and my jaw locked frequently. After just a week I have no pain and very minimal locking! I am so glad I came here to receive treatment for my TMJ and completely recommend their services as I have already improved so much!"

--Emma K.

"I'm feeling more rested when I wake up in the morning and have more energy throughout the day. During the night I am not as restless while sleeping and am able to get more comfortable in bed. My husband says I'm no longer snoring loudly, and he hasn't heard me gasping for air throughout the night. He also says I don't disturb his sleep anymore. I'm able to sleep with my bedroom door open because I'm sleeping quietly and not disturbing my daughter. I'm hoping to get healthier by having more energy to exercise."

--Kristen H.

"It was amazing how quickly wearing my mouth appliance took care of my jaw and ear pain! It takes a bit of getting used to but did not interfere with my daily life of talking especially, which I was worried about. As I'm into week 2, I'm working on increasing my ability to open which is improving every day. I can't say enough about how over the top friendly and helpful all the staff is and Dr. Patel as well."

--Mary F.

"My jaw used to click a lot, my jaw always locked, and was overall really uncomfortable and annoying. When I first came to Dr. Patel, he was able to immediately pinpoint and find the problem and made a jaw appliance to help fix my jaw. 3 to 4 weeks after initial treatment, all jaw clicking and locking has stopped. Really simple and easy. Thank you Dr Patel & staff!!"

--Jacob R.

"TMJ disorder was a constant inhibiting factor in my day-to-day life. Headaches prevented me from concentrating or enjoying free time. Within weeks after being fitted for a TMJ device by Dr. Patel, my pain was near nonexistent, and my headaches completely gone. I'm so grateful I made this choice to get treatment from Dr. Patel's office."

--Emma K.

"When I came to see Dr. Patel, I was in a lot of pain and experiencing extreme dizziness. Dr. Patel and his staff were very helpful and made sure I understood everything they found out during the evaluation. They provided a game plan on day 1 and I walked out knowing there was something that could help relieve my symptoms I had for the last 9 months. I have been wearing my retainer for the last month and in that time, I have seen and experienced a significant improvement in my symptoms and pain. I am so grateful for all Dr. Patel and his staff have done for me this last month!"

--Brittany W.

"Within one week of wearing my appliance—no jaw pain, no jaw popping or clicking, no locking of my jaw. I anticipate continued progress by wearing the appliance."

--Lois C.